A LIFE LARGER THAN PAIN
THE PATHWAY FROM RESIGNATION TO RENEWAL

ERV HINDS, M.D.

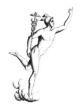

Health Press
Albuquerque, New Mexico

Published by Health Press
P.O. Box 37470
Albuquerque, NM 87176
www.healthpress.com

Library of Congress Cataloging in Publication Data

Hinds, Ervin A., 1941-
A Life Larger than Pain / by Erv Hinds
cm.
ISBN 0-929173-43-0

Design by Ruth Martin
Author photo by Mark Nohl
Cover photo by Ruth Martin

ACKNOWLEDGEMENTS

My sister, Ann Tull, encouraged me to expand a lecture on pain and spirituality into a book. She contributed to many aspects of this book, from the original vision to the final details. Thanks to her continued support I was able to complete this book while maintaining my professional practice.

Kathryn Helmers started as my agent, but evolved into my collaborator. Her literary skills helped me thread the philosophy and spiritual substance into the medical science matrix of the book, and her experience as an agent helped guide this book to publication.

My daughter, Emily Hinds, helped me refine my ideas into clear concepts. My niece, Linda Revol, worked extensively on researching the citations.

Friends and colleagues, Robin Hermes, M.D., Kevin Pauza, M.D., Kathryn Moore, and Jan Comeau, read the book and offered encouragement and direction.

Pastor Talitha Arnold, Sister Mary Joaquin, Terath Kaur Khalsa, Maria Matus, Carl Miller, Dan Namingha, Carolyn Silver, and Norman Yazzie shared their stories and spiritual paths.

DEDICATION

To my patients, from whom I have learned many of life's lessons as I watch them move from entrenchment in pain to renewal.

*Every experience opens the door
into a temple of new light,
although the vestibule may be dark and dismal.*

—ABRAHAM HESCHEL

CONTENTS

PREFACE

S O MANY THINGS in life turn out to be something entirely different than what they seemed at the outset. This is especially true of chronic pain and serious illness. The very thing we fear as a tragedy may be the springboard that jolts us out of spiritual complacency into profound growth.

Fifteen years ago, I was a young anesthesiologist planning ahead for the college education of three small children, running mini-marathons, and feeling somewhat smug about my success in life. Even though I had been a heart team anesthesiologist, I was ignoring my own loud heart murmur—at least subconsciously.

One day, feeling particularly tired after a ten kilometer race and needing an insurance policy exam, I had a chest x-ray. It revealed an enlarged heart, which was determined to be due to mitral valve insufficiency. Devastated by what was a life-limiting defect, I started the tortuous and frightening path to regaining health.

Close friends and a wise pastor helped me find the spiritual and psycho-logical strength to locate this solution across the Atlantic. In 1985, heart valve repair was not common in the United States, largely due to the steep learning curve in a severe medical and legal climate. Through research, prayer, and spiritual guidance from multiple sources, I chose to go to France and have my heart valve repaired by Dr. Alan Carpentier—a pioneer in heart valve repair.

I regained my health, but not without a shift in consciousness. I became more sensitized to a universal problem—that of pain and suffering.

I write this book as a man who has had a major change of heart, both literally and figuratively. I want to take readers on a journey of listening to the wisdom of my patients. But their experiences are ultimately your story and my story as well, for pain is not limited to physical injury or illness. Sooner or later, heartache from the loss of a relationship or the death of a loved one strikes us all. This is a poignant experience of pain, which I will also address in this book.

I am now a full-time doctor of pain medicine, after practicing anesthesiology for twenty-five years. Finally, I am doing what I went to medical school for—treating the whole patient, addressing the total pain experience. Paradoxically, I have become the student of my patients, learning daily how some meet adversity with spiritual expansion.

While treating the total pain experience it became apparent that encouraging patients to find their spiritual kernel was essential to redefining wellness. Much has been said about the body-mind connection in obtaining relief from pain, but I have observed that the body-mind-spirit connection is what gives purpose to a patient's pain. Many of my patients have revealed how their particular spiritual path has helped them reframe their life with pain. Many of them have found that pain has helped them redefine their beliefs, and they would not choose to return to a life without a spiritual center.

I have written down these thoughts and stories for the benefit of pain sufferers, their friends and loved ones, physicians, therapists, and even spiritual directors. My hope is to provide an understanding of the complexities of the pain experience; to encourage a deeper reverence for the integral unity of the human person—body, mind, and spirit; and to renew hope for a life no longer dominated and determined by pain. To stretch your thinking on pain and its various treatments, I will do more than present facts and observations. I will dramatize them in experience by telling stories to help you perceive the inevitable reality of pain in new and different ways. I will tell you some of my own stories, especially those responsible for my awakening as a healthcare provider and pain specialist.

I would like to give healthcare providers a degree of comfort in addressing spiritual issues as an integral part of treating pain patients. I want to help caregivers view the pain experience not as a dead end, but as a journey which may take surprising twists and turns in leading to a life that is enlarged rather than diminished by the intrusion of pain. And for all of you who are caught in the grip of pain, may you discover that what has threatened to undo you can become the harbinger of your wholeness.

At some bend in the road as we walk through life, all of us may experience the "pain paradox": *the very thing that is supposed to help you may make the pain worse, and what you think will hurt you may be the thing that frees you from a pain-dominated life.*

—Dr. Erv Hinds
Santa Fe, NM, September 2002

CHAPTER ONE

THE POWER OF PERCEPTIONS

The last resort of pain control strategies—altering the perception of pain—remains the most mysterious. The human mind is the most important and least understood arena of modern pain management. We all suffer from the same diseases and injuries, but we don't perceive them in the same way.

—DR. FRANK T. VERTOSICK, JR.[1]

THERE IS NO SUCH THING as life without pain. But for those in acute or chronic pain, there is no real life possible without some relief from its relentless punishment.

I am a pain doctor. My specialty is one of the most rapidly growing areas in medicine. The suffering individuals who walk through the door of our clinics come to us because their pain won't go away and they don't know where else to turn. For many of them, we are the last stop on a long journey of medical evaluations, procedures, and prescriptions. They are losing confidence in healthcare providers. They are losing hope.

A woman walks into our examining room for her initial appointment. She is a professional woman in her early fifties and CEO of her own successful business. She has worked hard to get where she is in life. She has done all the right things, and they have paid off. Just when she reaches the peak of her accomplishments and begins to enjoy her hard-earned satisfaction, she is struck with excruciating back pain. Her life has virtually come to a halt.

The problem began when she herniated a lumbar disc. Due to increasing weakness in her right leg, the neurosurgeon performed a disectomy. Unfortunately, she developed some scar tissue around nerve roots after the operation. This consequence led to a different but more severe pain than she had originally endured. In an attempt to alleviate this new pain, she underwent yet another surgical procedure. There was some temporary relief within a few weeks, but the pain came back again, this time in a slightly different pattern—nagging, constant, and lacerating. The problem just won't go away.

I can hear in the tone of her voice and see in the lines of her face that she is disillusioned and afraid. She has done all the right things, but they did not help her with her pain and suffering. In fact, she now has more intense pain, of a different quality, than she had prior to entering the healthcare system. Depression has set in; she has trouble sleeping; she cannot concentrate on her work as she once did; and she has no energy for relationships.

The pain seems to be taking over her life. She is worried about how she is going to keep her business going, because there is only so much she can delegate, and the stakes are high. But she is fresh out of medical and emotional resources for dealing with the pain. The surgeon who performed her back operations is out of ideas. There is nothing more he can do for her, she is told. She is angry at the feeling that others simply expect her to get over it. In fact, she suspects that some think it's all in her head. This is especially frustrating for a woman who has spent her adult life priding herself on her clear-headed realism. It is humiliating to feel that she is perceived as a hypochondriac. She didn't get this far in life by feeling sorry for herself or making up problems—quite the opposite. But the pain is beyond her control, and no matter what it only gets worse. As a last resort, she has been referred to the Pain Center in Santa Fe.

During our initial visit, in the process of listening to her story and performing a thorough neurologic and physical exam, I become convinced that her pain is all too real and her depression profound. I conclude that placing a needle at the scarred nerve and injecting anti-inflammatory medication under x-ray guidance (a transforaminal epidural) might alleviate some of her pain temporarily. It might also down-regulate the pain cycle, which would quiet the pain messages that her body is transmitting back and forth between the site of the problem and the brain. In the long term, however, it is clear to me that my mission is to help her open up to some psychological, behavioral, and eventually spiritual resources that may expand what she now considers very contracted options.

In order to accomplish this mission, my initial challenge at the outset is to give her a sense of hope—a tiny thread of inner renewal she can grasp hold of as we start our journey together. For her, I will play a new role as a medical practitioner: not a fix-it specialist who cures her problem, but a facilitator who helps her catalyze her own powers of healing. I will help her rethink her current circumstances, reframe her pain, and learn to draw upon her own inner resources. She is not even aware of these resources right now, because her perspective is so cramped by the incessant pain and its accompanying discouragement.

My goal in this initial visit is that when she walks out the door, she will feel that far more has taken place than the fatiguing routine of yet one more physical examination. I want her to be touched beyond the merely physical routine of examining symptoms and gathering data. I want her to have a much different experience than what she has been conditioned to anticipate from the medical establishment.

I know this woman will have to face the reality that although there is a great chance of healing, there may not be a cure. She will evolve, but it will be frightening to leave the concept of cure behind—the assumption that there is a procedure or medicine or shot out there somewhere that will entirely eliminate her problem. We have a long road ahead to walk together. But I know that as she lets go of her hopes for being cured and moves toward the truth of the realities she must live with, the process will catapult her into emotional and spiritual growth beyond her previous expectations. She will have a new and different energy for her work and her relationships as she evolves into healing of the mind and heart, even though it may not entail the physical restoration she has been seeking.

THE PROBLEM THAT WON'T GO AWAY

The lead article in *U.S. News and World Report*, March 17, 1997, was titled "The Quality of Mercy. Effective pain treatments already exist. Why aren't doctors using them?"[2] The writer cited the staggering costs of unrelieved suffering: 34 million people in the country suffer from chronic pain. Each year, millions seek relief at hospitals or pain clinics. Back pain, migraine, and arthritis rack up medical charges amounting to $40 billion annually. Chronic pain accounts for one-fourth of all sick days taken—50 million lost work days.

The American Academy of Pain Medicine estimates that pain costs the American people $120 billion each year.[3] Only one-third of persons suffering with chronic headaches seek treatment. Nearly 90 percent of all diseases are manifested through pain.

The experience of pain is a reality for every human being. It will happen to each of us: today, tomorrow, years from now in the aging process, or through the suffering of a loved one. Biologically, pain is a virtual certainty—as universal as eating and sleeping.

One in five Americans currently lives with chronic pain. At least 14 percent of these sufferers have headaches severe enough to miss work and to qualify them for some disability. Millions of Americans have low back pain or pain associated with whiplash, Herpes zoster, peripheral neuropathies, cancer, or with chronic diseases such as AIDS, diabetes, and arthritis.

I propose that we rethink how we approach pain, how we try to alleviate it, and how we understand it. I would like to question our conventional assumptions and responses by exploring how much they are influenced by cultural values we have uncritically assimilated. I want to point out that over time, and across other cultures, this problem has been dealt with in very different ways—and, in many cases, more creatively and effectively than in our current society, which seems to focus narrowly on the goals of pleasure and immediate gratification. Within the borders of our own country, there is enough cultural diversity and richness to offer significant opportunities for cross-cultural observations of the differences in how various ethnic groups and religious traditions deal with the problem of pain.

For all those who at the most common level share the experience of vulnerability to pain, I hope to awaken the thought that pain is not simply a negative physiological and psychological response to injury. Because pain has been with us since childhood as an inevitable and regularly occurring fact of life, we are so close to it that we cannot see the forest of meaning beyond the trees. We respond rather than reflect. We flee rather than find reason to stay within the moment and understand more deeply this very universal human experience.

OUR PAIN PHOBIA

As Americans have progressed into more pleasure and less discomfort, our comfort zones have narrowed considerably. Two generations ago, before air conditioning and central heating systems, people experienced the seasonal changes of temperature extremes and lived with discomfort as part of daily life. Severe cold or heat was simply a part of the cycle of nature. Now, our technology has enabled us to insulate ourselves from extremes. We like our indoor temperature to hover around 73°-74° F, and only a utility crisis will get us to change it.

This accommodation to physical comfort is representative of the way our society deals with discomfort in general. We are out of practice in dealing with it on a daily basis. In our pleasure-seeking society, we are less likely to bump up against the ordinary hardships and privations our great-grandparents took for granted. We have no idea that there may even be some pleasure outside the comfort zone.

Our society is pain-phobic as well as aging-phobic. We tend to associate pain with deterioration and aging—a process our culture fears rather than honors. But the best way to disarm fears about terminal illness and possibilities of great pain is to face them in advance, to prepare for them, and to think about death as a naturally-occurring part of life. Aside from grieving personal loss and sharing others' grief in community, one of the reasons we go to funerals may be our psychological need to prepare for death. The proliferation in recent years of books on death and dying reflects the dearth of ways our society offers for preparing and undergoing this universal experience.

In the United States, advertising feeds our dependence as consumers by conditioning us to believe that staying healthy is a complicated matter beyond the grasp of the average person. We are obsessed with maintaining physical health, as if vitamin supplements, carefully calibrated exercise, the perfect blend of herbal remedies, pain killers, and a trillion dollars annually invested in medical expertise are necessary to prop up our fragile existence. I wonder if most of us would do just as well by practicing periods of solitude, silence, and simplicity.

In Western society we tend to speak about body, mind, and spirit as separate categories. In the last few decades there has been a trend toward holistic integration of these components of the human person, largely because we have treated them in isolation from one another. In Santa Fe, where I live, the communal melting pot is strongly flavored by Native American cultures. Compartmentalizing existence is alien to Native Americans, who view such Western fragmentation with wry amusement. To them, reality is all one, and everything in life has a spiritual basis. Body and mind are not spoken of independently from the spirit.

The Native American's spirituality is the entire matrix for their existence. They see this spirituality in animals, trees, and nearly everything that goes on in life. The processes of body and mind follow naturally from the spirit, at the center of this matrix. Pain is not an alien and fearful enemy but a natural dimension of life in this world, an aid in preparing for life in the next world.

SHIFTING PERSPECTIVE

Medical sociologist M. H. Becker speaks about the new cult of physical fitness, diet, and maintaining one's best chance for health.[4] The current emphasis in healthcare promotion is risk reduction, self-discipline, and motivation to attain health. Becker says this new focus fosters a dehumanizing self-concern that substitutes personal health goals for more important human society goals. It is a new religion in which we worship ourselves, attaining the nirvana of good health through disciplined devotion to diet and exercise. Illness is punishment.

This new religion of individualism emphasizes health spas, beauty aids, the ideal diet, and the perfect combination of herbs—the pursuit of a narcissistic self-actualization at the expense of a better balance with spirituality, with community, and with relationships. Adherents to this religion are especially unprepared to face the trials of disease and deterioration. All their hard work in observing the dos and don'ts has led not to the promised immunity from suffering, but to the bitter taste of defeat.

Our technological age has bred in us a preoccupation with technique and created the illusion that we are in control of our lives. It has fed our sense of entitlement to long life and physical beauty. Ancient wisdom recognized the shortcomings of such a perspective. "No man can have a peaceful life who thinks too much about lengthening it," cautioned the Roman philosopher Seneca. A Latin proverb asserts, "He who lives medically lives miserably." The rapid trend toward specialization in medicine has brought disadvantages along with benefits. Attention has shifted from the person to the body parts: instead of treating a whole human being, we diagnose ailments in discrete organs, systems, and functions. Patients are left to sort out conflicting opinions and batteries of procedures without much help in sizing up the whole picture or integrating a bewildering array of data.

Medical fragmentation has carried over into pain management, one of the newest specialties in the medical establishment. Pain medicine integrates a mechanistic, technique-oriented approach with mind-body practices to complement localized treatment of specific pain sites. But the unique suffering of those in chronic pain affects them in all areas of life—physical, mental, and emotional. Managing this suffering rather than succumbing to it requires cultivating inner strength and developing a transcendent framework of understanding.

Along with the development of penicillin and the polio vaccine, the most significant medical advances of the past century include the twelve-step approach to treating addictions. The Alcoholics Anonymous (AA) movement has had a profound influence in helping millions of people to become functional members of society again. Although it is spiritually based, it uses concepts and language that include a wide spectrum of belief and unbelief in a divine being while affirming a reality that transcends the individual. Stepping outside one's own framework is crucial, because self-deception is what keeps the addict from recognizing and managing addictive behavior. By affirming the need for a greater power within a supportive group therapy setting, the AA program frees people to look beyond themselves and embrace powerful opportunities for healing.

The recovery movement blossomed as alcoholics discovered that through this experience of pain and suffering, their lives became more meaningful than they had been before the onset of the addiction, because the consequent personal growth extended into all aspects of life. In this process of overcoming, many individuals discover new and untapped potential.

Entrenchment in chronic pain is not unlike alcohol dependency in that sufferers are consumed by a concentration on self—specifically, they are fixated on the body. The technical term for this is "somatically-focused." If pain patients can get outside themselves by redirecting their focus onto a greater power, they can begin to break the stranglehold of their entrenchment.

Pain physicians can help entrenched chronic pain patients to focus beyond the body through interdisciplinary therapies. Behavioral psychology, physical therapy, and cognitive treatment—to name just a few—create fertile ground for a patient's individualized recovery process. They help individuals get outside the framework of their pain and view it from a distance, giving them the chance to see glimmers of color beyond the dark and gray world to which they have been confined.

In 1988, Dr. John Riley and his colleagues at Brown University studied the association of a chronic pain diagnosis with physical impairment (i.e., the inability to do certain kinds of work).[5] They found that many patients believe pain automatically implies impairment. Yet the bedrock of treatment for chronic pain—reactivation or increasing appropriate activity—is the opposite of impairment. Our society bombards us with quick-fix promises and miracle cures. We have been conditioned to look for something that will make the pain go away, fast. We associate pain with shutting down, not with increasing our levels of activity and mobility.

Effective treatment of acute and chronic pain generally requires a fundamental shift in perspective. It is not easy to change your way of looking at life—advice and information alone are not enough for most of us to do the hard work of personal growth. My own greatest changes have come from the crises of major transitions and life-threatening events.

We might not be able to change the fact of pain, but we can change how we allow it to affect us. Most of us are not very good at doing this, because we have been acculturated with the expectation of a pain-free life.

REFRAMING REALITY

"As he recovers from chronic fatigue syndrome, Keith Jarrett produces a CD of simple grace," reported *Time* magazine in a profile of the jazz pianist.[6] For over two decades the internationally-renowned musician had cultivated a highly successful performance and recording career. Then he was stopped in his tracks by an illness that came on suddenly and would not go away. He entered a long night of suffering, unsure if the day would ever dawn when he could play again.

After two years he began making improvements, but they were painfully slow. "Basically, I can't do my work," he told *Time* reviewer Terry Teachout. "But I'm doing dribs and drabs of it. I can do a little more all the time." He began recording again in the effort to give his wife a Christmas present, so tired that he could manage only a few minutes per session. And then a miracle occurred. "Something started to click with the mike placement, the new action of the instrument—I could play *so soft*—and the internal dynamics of the melodies of the songs. It was one of those little miracles that you have to be ready for, though part of it was that I just didn't have the energy to be clever." The fatigue seemed to shift the center of his creativity from the intellectual to the intuitive. Jarrett described the event in the language of purification: "It's almost as though I was detoxing from standard chordal patterns. I didn't want any jazz harmonies that came from the brain instead of the heart."

This is a striking illustration of a reversed perspective on pain: from an enemy that shuts down options to a catalyst for new directions. Although we would not wish such an agent of change on anyone, we can celebrate what emerges from the suffering. "Rarely has a jazz album come so directly from the heart," raved Teachout. Chronic fatigue changed the way Keith Jarrett played his music, and something new and lovely came from it.

Reframing reality involves letting go of previously held expectations of what life would be like. This is a painful and difficult process. But it contains the seeds of hope, because it nurtures openness to what may be given to us in the present. From the ashes of dashed hopes, new ideas and hidden gifts may emerge. Some gifts are all the more precious because they are unexpected.

Those in constant pain don't have the luxury of ignoring the difficult lessons of life. Because they are forced to live outside their comfort zone, they have an opportunity to glimpse what lies behind the veil of everyday reality. For some, this will be a sense of eternity, renewing their perspective on the here-and-now. For others, it may be confronting head-on the issues of personal growth they have been avoiding, or changing priorities while there is still time to focus on what ultimately matters.

*   *   *

At the end of our initial consultation, my new patient leaves with a prescription for temporary pain-relief and another appointment. Next time we will explore cognitive skills for dealing with pain, such as biofeedback, hypnosis, and relaxation. I will discuss with her some ways in which she can gradually become physically active again, both in working around the pain and in working through it. We will review the anatomy and physiology of her pain problem, so that she understands what kinds of procedures might decrease, or down-regulate, her pain. And I will begin listening for her spiritual kernel.

Later that day while driving home, I remember the desperate look on her face when she said to me, "Doctor, the pain just keeps getting worse. What am I going to do?" I counteract her despair by visualizing the opportunity I have to help her. In the process of facilitating her transition from raw pain and suffering to personal and spiritual growth, I will watch her learn to celebrate her uniqueness. If we are successful, what loomed as defeat will lead to renewal. This is the paradox at the heart of the pain experience.

I am choosing to take the journey of transformation with my patient. I know there may be periods of marked discouragement and disappointment for her. The threat of failure will weigh heavily on me as well. Physicians are as ego-driven as anyone else, and it would be much easier to practice in a more concrete, cause-and-effect environment—when someone has appendicitis, you take the appendix out. The before-and-after with an appendectomy is clear, and it feels much better than persevering through the uncertainties of discovering which drug may help and which procedure will promise a benefit outweighing the risk. But with tenacity and divine guidance, I trust that together she and I will walk through and overcome the obstacles of discouragement and frustration.

It is exciting for me to see patients evolve, each in a profoundly unique way, beyond their pain and suffering. It's like watching the desert bloom after a rain, changing immediately from a desolate landscape to one of surprising luminescence. My job is to help pain sufferers move beyond the cramped confines of a life constricted by pain to arrive at a new sense of wholeness. Each time this happens, it is a sacred event. Our Western culture tends to view pain as a mechanical problem—diagnose the origin of the injury and apply scientific expertise to eliminate the cause or repair its results. But the process of transformation extends beyond the physical plane. The most significant work I do as a pain doctor takes place where the limits of technological expertise meet the power of the human spirit.

STEPS FOR THE PATH:
EVALUATE YOUR PERCEPTIONS OF PAIN

To help you experience what you are reading, an interactive section—containing self-test exercises, questions for reflection, and suggestions to help strengthen body, mind, and spirit for pain relief—follows each chapter. You may find it helpful to use a separate journal or spiral-bound notebook as a place to record the steps you take along the path to a larger life. In addition to recording responses to questions at the end of each chapter, try writing in your journal frequently . Record what a good day is like and what a bad day is like. Observe any initiatives you made to manage pain, and when it seemed that the pain was managing you.

Choose a minimum level of regular entries, such as simply rating your pain on a scale of one to ten each day. This step alone can give you a sense of accomplishment in moving forward, helping to offset the sense of being trapped or stuck. When you look back across days and weeks, you may notice helpful patterns. Write them down.

If you are inclined to do so, pray about the steps you take to move from entrenchment to renewal. Consider asking a friend to encourage you by meeting with you regularly to talk about how you are doing with the Drag-Down Ds (see chapter two). Tell your doctor or healthcare provider what you're doing and what you're learning from it.

---

1. *Today, I would rate my general pain level as:*

    0   1   2   3   4   5   6   7   8   9   10
    pain free   excruciating pain

2a. *Use the statements on the next page to help you evaluate how your pain affects your general well-being. For each statement, check the box for the response that is most true for you.*

	always	usually	sometimes	seldom	never
I feel a sense of hope for the future.	☐	☐	☐	☐	☐
I have a strong sense of self-worth.	☐	☐	☐	☐	☐
I have confidence in my ability to accomplish the tasks of everyday living.	☐	☐	☐	☐	☐
I am generally satisfied with the quality of my relationships.	☐	☐	☐	☐	☐
I am able to take responsibility for my own wellness.	☐	☐	☐	☐	☐
I can take initiative in pursuing alternatives to drugs for managing my pain.	☐	☐	☐	☐	☐
I feel a sense of wholeness and purpose in my life.	☐	☐	☐	☐	☐

2b.   *Review your answers to the chart above. What are the most significant ways in which your pain shapes your attitudes and perspectives?*

3.   *Do you agree or disagree that changing your perceptions of pain can change your experience of pain?*

CHAPTER TWO

DEFEATING THE DRAG-DOWN DS

*Sometimes I go about pitying myself
while I am carried by the wind across the sky.*

—CHIPPEWA SONG[7]

As I GET TO KNOW a patient after the initial visit, the pattern of entrenchment in chronic pain becomes apparent. In addition to listening for the anatomical location of pain, I watch for signs of clinical depression. Classic symptoms include declining activity level; loss of hope for the future; and low energy level for work, recreation, and relationships. A person consumed by pain has a very contracted view of life: virtually all aspects are darkly colored by his perceptions of his pain experience.

I have developed a checklist of these symptoms that I call the "Drag-Down Ds," and I ask patients to journal about them on a daily basis. Talking about what this exercise reveals is by far the single most helpful cognitive interaction I have found. As they reflect honestly on their attitudes and behavior, their perception of their entrenchment changes, and they begin to see new avenues for escaping this downward cycle of intensifying pain.

Virtually every person who comes into the pain center has one or more of this constellation of factors. Each time I begin listing them, patients recognize themselves immediately: depression, deactivation, dependency, doctor-seeking, drug-seeking, deteriorating relationships, and dormant spirituality.

Depression. Birtually all pain patients with chronic pain report depression and its effects on them. Cardinal signs are: loss of energy, deteriorating sleep patterns, and sadness over losses associated with the effects of pain.

Deactivation. Chronic pain patients lose motivation and energy for remaining active, whether in sports, at work, or at home with family. They're no longer doing what they want to do. It is an insidious deteriorating physical condition associated with weight loss or weight gain and muscle atrophy. Life has changed to a sedentary, slow rhythm.

Dependency. To compensate for the pain-induced limitations, patients are forced to rely on significant others, family members, and work colleagues to do simple or complex tasks that are really the responsibility of the pain sufferer. This dependency has a dampening effect on their self esteem.

Doctor-seeking. Patients frequently are seeking yet another doctor to help them with their chronic pain. They have a lurking feeling that if they can just find the right healthcare provider, a cure is in the offing.

Drug-seeking. Whether they want narcotics to blanket the pain or just a medication to help ease it, most pain patients are looking for more or different drugs. In desperation, pain sufferers find they are dominated and controlled by medications to relieve pain.

Deteriorating Relationships. Almost all people in chronic pain can point to close relationships that are now faltering or are less satisfying than they were prior to their entrenchment. The energy to nurture friendships is missing. Moodiness and irritability interfere with interactions with those close to them. Obsessive focus on health problems puts off family and friends.

Dormant Spirituality. Pain sufferers will often put their spiritual quest on hold while intensively seeking moments of pain relief. Few individuals who seek help for pain engage in a regular spiritual practice. Those who have developed faith convictions often experience severe testing of their beliefs under pressure of the health crisis. If patients can revive a dormant kernel of spiritual meaning, it will often open a new way forward through the pain.

Beginning to correct any of the Ds will break the downward spiral and start the process of change for all of them—a way back from dysfunctional, de-railed, and dealt-a-bad-deck-of-cards entrenchment. It begins to acknowledge the misconception that one is mired in a helpless, hopeless situation from which there is no escape.

A spiritual resurgence may be the only way to change this fatalistic attitude. Perhaps this is because fundamentally, no matter how body-based its triggers may be, despair is a collapse of the spirit. The perceived losses simply become too great to bear. The way back from such a collapse must involve a renewal of the spirit, not just treatment of the body.

When patients lose hope they tend to stop coming to the pain center, retreat into a reclusive lifestyle, and try to medicate their pain away. One of my patients doesn't go out of her house, has her food delivered, and focuses entirely on taking the medication, which has put her into a rebound problem. I explain to her that we are trying to get her off the medication and introduce warm water therapy, reactivation, and socialization—i.e., getting her out of the house and back into a social environment. But I sense that all she wants is for me to continue supplying the medication. She is fixated on it.

Despair, a living death, often conquers the spirit gradually, as hope is repeatedly withdrawn. But it is not inevitable. For some, ill health presents a special temptation. It is almost enjoyable to wallow in chronic pain, because it can yield secondary benefits such as attracting extra attention or providing an excuse for not acting responsibly. The remedy is to purge self-pity and divert attention from concern about the illness. But renouncing self-pity requires a new and not-so-cozy view of pain, because it may involve giving up a difficult luxury.

Relinquishing self-pity requires us to find resources of strength from within. This is the realm in which we learn to accept suffering without being defeated by it. Cancer patients nearing death will sometimes experience a deep inner peace as despair gives way to hope for the release of suffering, for the journey of the spirit out of the broken body to a home they sense is waiting for them.

AVOIDING WOUNDOLOGY

Dr. Carolyn Myss, author of *Why People Don't Heal and How They Can*, coined the term "woundology" to describe a self-perpetuating and obsessive focus on one's personal problem. However real the problems may be, there is a seductive power to the wound. The downside of the recovery movement is that the sharing of wounds has become "the new language of intimacy."[8] Myss observes that people confuse "the therapeutic value of self expression with permission to manipulate others with their wounds."[9]

Woundology is a very important concept for pain patients. A significant percentage of them want to talk about their victimization. This is different than processing wound issues in a healthy way, in which the goal is to move from preoccupation with the injury to recovery and health. Victimization vocabulary is peppered with words designed to draw attention to wounds, suffering, and difficult circumstances. They are perhaps unaware that they have created relationships and dependence problems surrounding their wounds. American society is fascinated with the wounds of post-traumatic-stress syndrome, sexual abuse, and workers' compensation injuries. These are critically important issues, and I don't intend to devalue them in any way—but our focus on these violations can foster unhealthy preoccupation with them.

The media has been at the forefront of dramatizing personal trauma and encouraging woundology discussions. This is just one example of how our society tends to feed on the wounded. Some attorneys routinely advertise to encourage people to seek money for their personal injuries and to stay wounded at least until there is some monetary reward for their wounds. Caroline Myss calls woundology "a kind of welfare state of the soul, paying people dividends for blithely refusing to better their condition."[10]

Penelope Johnson was a patient who came to me with victimization and the vocabulary of woundology so imbedded in her person that it was difficult to help her begin to heal or move beyond her pain and suffering. I first saw Penelope about three years ago, when she was referred to me for low back pain radiating into her legs. You could say she was a "larger than life" personality: rather attractive, very theatrical, quite intelligent, and markedly obese.

The treatment we chose, which Penelope complied with, was non-narcotic pain medication and a swimming program, in addition to consultation with a psychologist and group therapy. As I began to know Penelope better, she revealed to me that she was the "family secret." She had been sexually abused by her grandfather. Tragic as this was, it seemed to have an almost seductive effect in its power to make her feel special. With increased visits, the focus was not so much on the low-back pain and its radiation down the leg, but on her victimization.

Penelope told me that during her group therapy, patients talked about their early-life traumas. I asked what she thought could help people move beyond their wounds to growth, and she was appalled that anyone could see beyond this point. Had anyone discussed the power of forgiveness, I asked her, or how adversity can catapult people into different careers or onto new spiritual paths? Her only response was that she couldn't imagine how anyone could not talk about "the thing that is most important to all of us—our childhood injuries."

I later found out from Penelope's swimming instructor that her particular swim class spent at least half their time at the side of the pool talking about the problems that had brought them there, rather than swimming. Penelope would also appear occasionally with her walker or her crutches. The padding at the stem of the crutches or on the walker would be decorated with something seasonally appropriate—green shamrocks for St. Patrick's Day or red hearts for Valentine's Day, drawing even more attention to the physical disability.

Penelope tended to fire her family practitioners as they became less interested in her "family secret" and tried to address her problems directly. She sought out other physicians. She didn't like their failure to listen to her, and she would go in search of other physicians who would. When I introduced words such as forgiveness or tried to help her change her vocabulary of victimization, Penelope grew angry and told me that I had lost interest in her as a patient. Her efforts shifted to attempts to control the medications I was giving her.

We reached a point at which I felt it necessary to have a conference with Penelope and her family in which I talked very specifically about the value of letting go of injuries and suffering from the past, and formulating new goals. Change is not cozy, I told them. It can increase pain intensifiers such as fear and anxiety. But it can also increase pain inhibitors, such as hopefulness, which would help Penelope move through the transitions on a path away from self-pity toward self-reliance.

The result of this approach was Penelope's disappearance from my practice for at least a year. Then Penelope surfaced again, with the same problem, most likely after having consulted another pain center and repeating the same processes. This time I discussed with her the importance of spiritual renewal in breaking free of the victimization trap and moving beyond the self to spiritual growth. Penelope is now on a spiritual quest that is beginning to open some chinks in the armor of her woundology.

Many of my pain patients are trapped in their need to talk about their pains and wounds. They create relationships around their woundology, whether in the form of support groups or intimate attachments. It is important for pain sufferers to talk about their woundedness, but it is equally important for them not to get stuck there. In a society in which the media glamorize wounds and some systems reward victimization, it is difficult for many people to make any headway in getting past their obsession with hurt. Therefore, physicians and therapists are especially crucial in helping patients recognize this preoccupation as a dependency they need to work through rapidly in order to move toward healing. One of the most effective ways to do this is by turning things over to a higher source and strengthening the spiritual life. For some, it proves to be the only way to get beyond their "comfort with discomfort."

The opposite of woundology is empathy. Instead of focusing inward on one's own pain, an empathetic response recognizes that others are in the same or similar circumstances. Pain becomes the initiation into the fellowship of sufferers. Those who can help us most are those who understand our suffering because they have suffered themselves.

Ammachi, a Hindu saint, comes to Santa Fe about once a year. Ammachi, or Amma, is revered in India as a healer and sage. In her own country, she is widely known as the founder of large-scale social projects to help the poor through vocational training, to house battered women, to provide medical care in hospitals and hospices, to support orphanages, and to advance environmental causes. Around the world, she is know primarily as the saint with the "healing hug," freely offering love and compassion to all she meets.

"To show compassion to suffering humanity is our obligation to God," Ammachi believes. "The spiritual quest begins with selfless service to the world. In the yoga tradition, we cultivate dispassion, so we can meet death or pain fearlessly and without regret. You may not be able to renounce things easily, but you should try to quiet your mind." In the Hindu tradition, reincarnation brings the soul through successive lifetimes, "just as waves of an ocean appear in different forms and different sizes," and so Ammachi suggests that we face pain and death as if we're just working through another life. Instead of being preoccupied with our pain and fear, we can let go of self and extend empathy to others. "Those who dwell in a selfless state are constantly in the mood to give," Ammachi describes. "Gifts of the spirit pour from them continually. They are too busy giving to ask for anything in return."[11]

Woundology is the result of staying trapped in pain; empathy is one result of breaking out of the cycle of pain. The first is cultivated by a shallow absorption with self; the second, by a deep and abiding attention to the larger life of human community and spiritual reality.

SEEKING HARMONIOUS INTEGRATION

When responding to illness or trauma, it is tempting to withdraw into a cocoon of self-absorption, narrowing our vision to our own wounds as self-compassion devolves into self-pity in a downward spiral. By contrast, an integrated life is free from excessive and unhealthy preoccupation with self. It is structured in a way that permits integration of the self horizontally and vertically—personally, socially, and spiritually. The difference in these two responses to pain is the difference between the self in isolation and the self in harmony with its surroundings.

Our cultural background can predispose us to one response over the other. Under the pressure of pain, this predisposition is magnified. Our consumer culture tilts us toward the self-centered life, away from a communally-based life. It bombards us with the message, "You have the right to go after anything you want. You deserve the best that life has to offer." Pain is an unwelcome interruption of the pursuit of success, like experiencing a car breakdown on the highway. You tow the car to the nearest garage, fix the problem, and get back on the road to the good life as quickly as possible. In conventional medicine, illness is perceived mechanistically—a biological problem with biological and chemical remedies. Medication is the most time-efficient way to eliminate such an intrusion.

By contrast, both in traditional Hispanic medicine and for most Native Americans of the Southwest, physical illness is perceived as a violation of spiritual law. Healing is therefore imbued with the divine. Most *curanderas* (Hispanic faith healers) of the Southwest emphasize the association of sin and illness, because their cultural traditions have been strongly influenced by a mystical Catholicism. For Native Americans, healing involves the recovery of harmony and balance in human community embedded in the mysterious flow of nature. To lose that balance and harmony is to be in a wasteland of emptiness.

In each of these cultures, there is a confidence level operating that empowers healing. Native Americans see the healing power in nature and have confidence that it will combat illness. The curandera helps reinforce confidence in prayer to saints, in confession, and in doing penance. By contrast, our consumer culture leaves us vulnerable to a failure of confidence in healing when we reach the limits of our resources of scientific theory, technology, and pharmacology.

I like to use the words "tradition" and "trust" in discussing the social and cultural assumptions we bring to the pain experience. The Western tradition of healing has been based in medication and surgery, and therefore we trust that approach. When Catholics go to Lourdes for healing, they have trust in their religious tradition. Navajos put faith in the repetitive chanting of their "sing" man.

I have been very intrigued with the Navajo concept of harmony, because it models an integration that pain patients often lack, isolated from the normal routines of the rest of society. I interviewed a Navajo named Norman Yazzie, who works in the operating room at St. Vincent Hospital in Santa Fe. He is from a traditional family in Teec Nos Pos, Arizona. Several of his older family members do not speak English; his grandmother is a foremost Navajo rug weaver.

As Norman recounted Navajo ideas about birth, death, pain, and suffering, he emphasized that these life processes are integrated easily into the Navajo way. The essence of Navajo culture is the maintenance of hózhó, which means balance and harmony. To restore hózhó and to treat disease, the Navajo employs ancient healing ceremonies called the Chant Ways. Each Way involves a singer and sometimes a sand painting. Peyote priests and medicine people help those in pain and suffering to focus their attention away from the intense reality of pain toward the spiritual world.

In the Navajo concept of balance and harmony, there is no coincidence or accident. All of life, both positive and negative, has synchronicity. Things happen positively as a reward for living well spiritually. Things happen negatively as a consequence of imbalance with nature. Pain, suffering, and healing are all intrinsically woven into the balanced unity of life. The Navajo see human beings as so connected with the earth that illness is often traced to some interaction with nature.

Norman recalled being run through a gauntlet of tests for severe pain with a bladder infection when he worked at Jackson Hole Hospital in Wyoming. After suffering an allergic reaction to a radiological dye, he decided he was through with Western doctors. Much to their dismay, he got dressed and left for the Navajo reservation.

Treatment at the reservation involved herbs and healing ceremonies. With assistance from peyote priests and medicine people, Norman reconnected with Mother Earth and experienced a healing of his illness. The doctors were amazed when he came back to work pain-free. During the ceremony, Norman had been given a specific vision of a childhood incident in which he had offended the creatures of the earth. He felt that the bladder infection was a consequence, and it had been necessary to heal this wound and exorcise the pain. "We are so connected to the earth that when one offends nature there will be consequences," he concluded.[12]

Navajo approaches to health and healing are all deeply rooted in the earth. Their medicinal remedies involve herbs, gifts from Mother Earth. Eating corn pollen is a healing act with spiritual significance, because corn is related to creation. Eating deer and elk meat confers the strength of these muscular animals upon the humans who ingest them, appealing to the slain animals' spirits for renewal. Traditionally, pain is always dealt with from a spiritual standpoint, reflecting the harmony and balanced unity of all of life.

The fragmented nature of Western culture works against pain patients. Chronic pain usually narrows the victim's world. It takes so much energy to fight the pain, there is little energy for other people and expanding personal horizons. Sincere attempts from others to extend care often fall short of what is needed. Instead of authentic presence and compassion, people will sometimes toss off shallow statements such as, "I know how you must feel." These expressions often have the effect of further isolating the sufferer. Yet it is imperative for people in chronic pain to avoid isolation. The burden of suffering can be eased in the context of healthy relationships that help to give the pain patient a sense of worth and identity that is defined by caring people, not by the limitations of the pain.

ACCEPTING OPPORTUNITIES FOR GROWTH

Sometimes adversity can be viewed as a purification—a sifting process in which the winds of difficult change sweep away the chaff to reveal the wheat that is worth harvesting. In this process, whether inaugurated by the onset of chronic pain or through deliberate submission to a spiritual discipline, there is usually an increase in stress and internal conflict before any transformation takes place.

If life is smooth and you are relatively free of physical and emotional pain, you are much more likely to swim with the flow of the surrounding culture. It will be difficult not to hunger for more power and money. But if you are in constant pain, you will find it very difficult to feel successful by conventional standards. When you are struggling, the likelihood of inward change is much greater.

Chronic pain sufferers have been given a difficult gift of accelerating the process of inner growth. They have a chance to move on to a transformation of character and perspective, to see the world with new eyes and a new heart. In the New Testament epistle to the Romans, the apostle Paul described transformation as a change from being conformed to earthly things to being enlightened by the power of the Spirit.[13] Another way to describe this change is a shift from being outer-directed to becoming inner-directed: from being shaped by the superficial demands of a consumer culture to making choice based on personal convictions of what is ultimately important.

Instead of viewing struggle as a setback or personal defeat, we can choose to see it as a window opening on a new view of the world— perhaps even a glimpse of the eternal. When earthly life seems to be fleeting and fragile, we naturally turn to what is of lasting value. The longer we are forced to stay within the struggle, the greater our opportunity to forge a new way of looking at life and new ways of being in the world. This response to the challenge of pain is a marvelous choice to move toward growth rather than passively accept stagnation.

In the process of overcoming adversity, some people break through to astonishing new levels of growth. Athletes such as Lance Armstrong, the cyclist who overcame a near-fatal battle with testicular cancer and went on to win the Tour de France four times, came back from crippling blows to reach heights of accomplishment no one thought possible. Great leaders have often suffered great adversity—Abraham Lincoln endured severe depression for much of his adult life; polio left Franklin Roosevelt in a wheelchair. Pain and suffering can motivate people to go far beyond their comfort zones in the commitment to hope for a better life.

*　　　*　　　*

Eric Varella, a big man who used to be a very good athlete, developed significant and chronic neck pain after his car was rear-ended. He was a conscientious employee and continued to work at his job as an auto mechanic. The pain was severe and constant, however, severely limiting the range of motion in his neck. He developed a pattern of depression, dragged-down relationships, and some deactivation. Since he had drifted away from his Catholic upbringing, he would need to find a way to rekindle his spiritual strength.

We emphasized Eric's need to begin the process of reactivation. He began swimming on a regular basis, but the neck pain persisted. Determined to decrease the pain, we performed xray-guided proce-dures—a cervical epidural followed by cervical facet (joints in the neck) injections. Now Eric was able to move his neck with less pain and his headaches decreased in intensity and frequency. Through two years of struggle, he learned that his adversity created an opening for him to rebuild his spiritual life. As he re-entered the Catholic Church, he began moving from depression to hope. His inward renewal, combined with physical reactivation, is helping him function more effectively and with less pain. His is not a welcome situation, but at times it is a joyful one.

Responding to pain with despair and withdrawal leads to entrenchment and woundology. Responding to pain with determination to discover a larger life leads to hope. Both involve suffering, but they lead in very different directions.

STEPS FOR THE PATH:
IDENTIFY YOUR ENTRENCHMENT

1. *Today, I would rate my general pain level as:*

    0   1   2   3   4   5   6   7   8   9   10
    pain free   excruciating pain

2a. *To assess the degree of your entrenchment in pain, use the following scale to identify where you are on a continuum from the Drag-Down Ds to recovery from pain (a "10" represents the most positive position on the scale).*

    0   1   2   3   4   5   6   7   8   9   10
    depression   hope for the future

    0   1   2   3   4   5   6   7   8   9   10
    deactivation   reactivation

    0   1   2   3   4   5   6   7   8   9   10
    dependency   self-reliance

    0   1   2   3   4   5   6   7   8   9   10
    doctor-seeking   responsibility for my wellness

    0   1   2   3   4   5   6   7   8   9   10
    drug-seeking   pursuing alternatives

    0   1   2   3   4   5   6   7   8   9   10
    deteriorating relationships   renewed relationships

    0   1   2   3   4   5   6   7   8   9   10
    dormant spirituality   spiritually active

2b.   Reflect on the areas of your life in which you have the greatest opportunity to overcome entrenchment and move toward renewal.

3.   Imagine that you are reviewing yourself on video. How and when do the Drag-Down Ds show up in your behavior?

CHAPTER THREE

Pain Does Not Equal Suffering

The thing that causes our suffering is also causing our endurance,
which is bringing us hope.

—ROBERT K. HUDNUT[14]

W E COMMONLY ASSUME that pain and suffering are virtually the same thing. But they need to be differentiated. Pain is the body's response to tissue injury—or, as with heartache, the spirit's response to emotional injury. Suffering is our emotional response to pain, whether from bodily hurt or heartache. However, not all suffering is experienced equally. In large part suffering is determined by cultural background, support systems, individual psychological makeup, and spiritual beliefs.

Specific research exists concerning cultural differences in pain, suffering, and spirituality. Some of it dates from 1965 by Harvard Medical School's Richard Sternbach and Bernard Tursky, who studied different responses to pain among old Americans of Protestant-British, Jewish, Italian, and Irish descent.[15] They discovered significant differences in the way Italian and Hispanic Americans outwardly respond to pain as compared with Protestant British Americans. This is awkward to discuss in our current climate of heightened sensitivity toward ethnic differences and racial minorities. But in fact, the way we are raised, our neurosignatures on our belief systems, and our remembered wellness do affect the way we respond to pain.

Such investigations are not intended to create and reinforce stereotypes. Rather, they suggest that pain is only pain as we know it. Our upbringing and our heritage contribute to our perception of pain, and therefore to our ability to endure it. They also influence our views of treatment, and whether we include or exclude spiritual belief and religious tradition in the ways we adjust to pain.

For example, guilt is frequently associated with pain. Images of a wrathful god bent on punishing wrongdoers haunt some sufferers, especially those from conservative or fundamentalist Judeo-Christian backgrounds. But guilt is counter-productive to helping us deal with and move beyond the physical and psychological immobilization resulting from chronic pain. Within the same religious traditions, there are role models of people who turned away from the burden of guilt and toward the power of prayer.

Pema Chödrön, an American woman who converted to Zen Buddhism, became a Tibetan nun and founded the Gampo Abbey in Cape Breton, Nova Scotia, the first Tibetan monastery in North America established for Westerners. In one of her books, *When Things Fall Apart: Heart Advice for Difficult Times*, she juxtaposes Western and Eastern ways of handling pain. One approach avoids it; the other "leans into it." The differences are profound. All of us naturally fear pain and try to avoid it at any cost. "Generally speaking, we regard discomfort in any form as bad news." We do not realize that the situations of pain and suffering are teaching moments. We automatically hate them and try to escape from them. "This very moment is the teacher."[16] For the Tibetan Buddhist, suffering is a given, one of the basic truths of life. The Westerner tries to avoid pain and suffering, swinging wildly between extremes of fear and hope instead of calmly accepting the impermanence of these temporal realities.

GOOD AND BAD SUFFERING

Most of us live in fear of suffering. In our American culture, it is the thing we try hardest to avoid. Pain must therefore be eliminated, because pain inevitably causes suffering, and we presume that suffering is always bad. It will deny us the life we want. It will be unbearable.

If we change our responses to pain, however, we can change the nature of our suffering even without eradicating the pain. We tend to think only a cure will do. In a few fortunate cases, a cure can be accomplished, eliminating the injury and the pain associated with it. But in many cases, a cure is simply not possible. What then?

Perhaps healing in its broadest sense means recovery from unbearable or meaningless suffering, which shuts us down and renders us unable to function. Physical recovery to some degree is necessary and important, but true healing encompasses psychological and spiritual restoration as well. To address healing—not just the reduction or elimination of pain—we must address all three dimensions of mind, body, and spirit.

I have strengthened my own spiritual foundations especially in seasons of change and crisis, when I have been forced to reevaluate everything in my life and identify what matters most in order to make wise choices. Although my path remains within the Christian tradition, I delight in learning from the wisdom of others' spiritual paths. I am privileged to work in a colorfully multicultural area of the country, where on a daily basis I am stimulated by the insights of those from other ethical and religious traditions. I have learned to value an authentic spiritual frame-work regardless of the specific teachings it comprises. This enables me to encourage my patients to draw from their own heritage or current convictions in developing a perspective that is larger than the pain consuming them.

I have witnessed again and again the centrality of one's spiritual perspective in breaking the destructive power of the pain cycle. Western medicine has grown increasingly sophisticated in its ability to pinpoint the causes of pain and develop highly specialized techniques for allevi-ating the pain. But even with this technological prowess, it is usually just palliative. It can dramatically change the level of pain, but unless it cures the problem by eliminating the injury, it cannot eliminate the pain entirely. Therefore, the patient remains vulnerable to the entrapment of the pain cycle. Breaking this cycle requires more than better technique.

How does one cope with pain when it cannot be eliminated? Certainly, by doing everything possible to minimize the pain and its effects. We continue to invest social resources heavily in accomplishing this goal. But just as important as coping with chronic pain—if not more important, given the now-documented benefits of spiritual approaches to physiological problems—is the transformation of suffering. It is possible to change our response to pain so that suffering has a redemptive effect, leading to a life larger than the pain, rather than a destructive effect that reduces life to the narrow confines of the pain. In our society, we know very little of such transformation. Many of us are not even aware that it is possible, because we are so distracted by the rush for immediate gratification in our attempts to escape pain and suffering. Yet for thousands of years, the great religious traditions have passed from one generation to the next their accumulated wisdom on this very subject.

I have often wondered why in this age of information we remain so short-sighted to the richness of our spiritual traditions in teaching us how to live, how to cope with infirmity, and how to die. In the past, these traditions have had power to shape existence just as effectively as our technologically advanced society—in some respects, even more so. Why do we feel that in the timeline of history, our brief minute on earth is where the answers will be found? Why do we not look back on the record of human experience with suffering, seeking with wonder and awe the insights of those who have endured pain and suffering and found wisdom to prevail with dignity—whether monks of medieval Europe, Native American healers, Tibetan Buddhists, or prisoners in concentration camps and the Gulag. We spend time and money on the latest trends while neglecting the richness of our spiritual traditions and their power to change our experience of illness, pain, and suffering. This is a tragic mistake.

In dealing with pain, we have opportunity to stand on the shoulders of those from past times and other cultures. I am not recommending that we all take courses in comparative religion and folk healing. Rather, I am suggesting that we get back in touch with whatever is authentic for each of us spiritually, taking time to reflect on what is ultimately important. The immediate-gratification impulse of our society shipwrecks on the shoals of pain.

In my work with patients—which involves what they teach me as much as my treatment of them—I have noticed a striking commonality in the diversity of religious traditions. I am no specialist in comparative religion, but the gathered wisdom of our spiritual teachers seems to converge in the difference between "good" and "bad" suffering—or what I would like to call redemptive versus destructive suffering. Those who remain trapped in the pain cycle suffer destructively. Those who break out of it suffer redemptively. One tears down the self and leads to further harm; the other builds up the self and leads to a new kind of wholeness. Each is based in a contrasting set of responses to pain. The power to choose between these responses depends on neither physical strength nor mental acuity. It lies in the province of the spirit. This is why spiritual resources are so absolutely vital to dealing with the problem of pain.

THE DIFFERENCE SPIRITUALITY CAN MAKE

Recognizing and acting on the spiritual dimension of pain can ease suffering instead of increasing it. This reality became clear in treating Isabel Lujan, an attractive, Hispanic woman who was thirty-five when she came to see me. Prior to an automobile accident the year before, she had been slim, athletic, and outgoing. Her personal charisma was matched by her keen intelligence. When the accident had occurred, it set off a complex of problems with her neck and lower back. She developed significant whiplash, resulting in chronic neck pain, headaches, and muscle (myofascial) pain.

For a year and a half Isabel had been going to a myriad of physicians and several orthopedic surgeons. She had been to neurologists and neurosurgeons for headaches and her other problems. All of them had looked at her body and done neurological examinations. They had evaluated her symptoms and prescribed very specific treatments. All this time she continued to have significant pain in her neck, arms, and one of her legs.

When Isabel came to me, I did a complete history and physical with a neurological examination and physical assessment. I also added her sleep history, family history, a history of what she used to like to do and what she can't do now, and a psychological evaluation. All this time her husband was part of the discussion.

I noticed that Isabel wore a crucifix around her neck. I asked her how she was managing, what it was that was helping her get through these difficult days of pain and lack of sleep. Prayer, she answered. We expanded on that subject and discussed her belief system. I asked if she would be willing to see a Catholic priest, who is also a Jungian psychologist, for guidance in dealing with discomfort and pain from a spiritual point of view. She said she would. Then we set out to make a plan about how to approach her pain and the crucial aspect of reactivation from being trapped in chronic pain. We discussed how to begin treating her sleep deprivation without narcotics or medications such as Valium. We began the process of examining her by doing different procedures that might give us some idea of how to treat her pain.

We discussed the importance of exploring cognitive-care principles. The dominant theme in her healing blueprint, however, was the intertwining of her spiritual belief system and exploring how her pain and suffering might increase her faith as well as her ability to help her family members.

Since that time I have seen Isabel once, and we have started her on medications to nudge her into better sleep. She is seeing the Jungian priest, and they have worked on some cognitive skills, meditation, hypnosis, and ways to integrate her spirituality into her suffering in a positive, effective way. We have begun to organize appropriate physical therapy and reactivation. The overall goal has been to give Isabel a sense of hope for the future and a new context for her chronic pain, involving her family, culture, and religious faith—a context that will help her turn her problem into a positive opportunity.

Sometimes adversity and pain initiate a process of purification—the unimportant or superfluous is drained off in the pressure of crisis, clarifying, and strengthening what remains. Classic patterns of spiritual purification suggest that there is always an increase of stress and a heightening of internal conflict before spiritual transformation takes place. Those in chronic pain have been given a difficult gift in the acceleration of this process.

If life is going well for you and physical or emotional pain is not an issue, it's easy to structure your life around the pursuit of success in conventional terms—career advancement, improving investments, getting more out of relationships and leisure time, planning vacations, and acquiring more sophisticated electronics. Perhaps this way of life is what the Apostle Paul was concerned with when he warned, "Do not be conformed to this world, but be transformed by the renewing of your mind."[17] It's very hard *not* to be hungry for power and money when you're successful.

In this age of specialization, we have become accustomed to separating the body into its distinct systems and organs and then hiring a specialist to diagnose and eliminate the problem. Yet no body part is an isolated organ or appendage, complete unto itself. Each is a part of the interconnected whole. I doubt that we will ever understand this unity completely.

Researchers have made tremendous strides in identifying the complexities of the mind-body relationship. The intricacies of brain and body invite respect and awe; the interrelation of mind, body, and spirit invites wonder. When pain attacks the body, it affects the mind and the spirit as well.

Yet studies show that epidemiology and spirituality remain distant strangers in much of conventional medicine. According to a poll, health professionals are far less religious than the general public. Nearly three-quarters of the U.S. population agreed with the statement, "my whole approach to life is based on religion," compared with only one-third of psychologists and under 40 percent of psychiatrists. Sixty-three percent believe it's good for doctors to talk to paitents about spiritual faith.[18]

David Larson, president of healthcare research for the National Institute of Health, states that less than one-half of one percent of published health research studies includes any basic variables of spiritual or religious commitment.[19] Studies that do take these variables into account show that despite medically-established bias to the contrary, over four-fifths of the general population associate religion and spirituality positively with both physical and mental health. Yet these religious variables are rarely discussed in professional medical networks, and clinicians and researchers continue to exclude religion from their work.

Education about spiritual variables, and openness to their potential role, can enable healthcare providers to become more effective healers. Some people tend to dismiss these variables as just another placebo—something with no scientific benefit, such as a sugar pill, that results in improvement. But even this simple phenomenon is a reminder that healing takes place that is not attributable to pharmacological ingredients or administered medical procedures. Perhaps the faith factor does at times function like a placebo—but it is different in a crucial respect: placebos almost always have a declining effect, but the faith factor can result in progressive and lasting improvement.

Growing interest in the interrelationships of spirituality, psychology, and health have put pressure on healthcare professionals to improve care by acquiring the necessary knowledge and skills to handle spiritual variables in practice. Some practitioners are skeptical of the value of religious beliefs simply because of their upbringing and personal experience. Others may oppose the mix of religion and medicine because of the dangerous risks of so-called faith healing; stories regularly hit the news of parents who refuse medical treatment for their children with preventable or curable illnesses. Nevertheless, physicians accept responsibility all the time to care for people who have habits and addictions they disapprove of or consider dangerous, such as alcoholism or heavy smoking. At the very least, they can accept the reality of a patient's belief system as one more factor in the mix. Compared to outright hostility or absolute avoidance, even such reluctant acceptance would be a step in the right direction.

There is a strong case to be made for the wisdom of healthcare professionals in practicing acceptance rather than judgment of a patient's spiritual beliefs. First, it is counter-productive to dismiss spiritual beliefs simply because of personal disinclination or distaste. At a basic level, that dismissal is really no different from indulging in dislike of an obese patient rather than endeavoring to understand the reasons for the obesity. Perhaps more importantly, however, discounting the potential of faith as a positive factor in wellness may very well withhold healing power from the patient.

Sometimes the spiritual dimension is neglected simply because we lack a common understanding of spirituality—it means so many different things to so many different people. For some, it has nothing to do with organized religion. For others, spirituality is defined by and inseparable from a specific religious system. The vast number of religious traditions and endless permutations of sectarian differences within them is confusing. And religious affiliation and belief tends to be viewed as a private matter, so that asking about it seems like an intrusion on intimately personal matters. Some professionals are wary of appearing to proselytize, especially when they are encountering people in a highly vulnerable state.

However, incorporating spirituality in medical care can be as simple and basic as treating those in pain and suffering with dignity. This is a way of affirming each individual as a whole human being, not simply a medical problem to be solved. I often tell patients going into the operating room that the O.R. staff is interested not just in their safety and comfort but in their dignity as well. Acknowledging their endurance of adverse circumstances is a way of honoring the whole person. When people are made to feel worthy of individual attention and respect, the severity of their pain tends to lessen. When they are not treated with dignity, suffering usually intensifies.

Honoring patients at their time of death is another way of acknowledging the human spirit. When we're very young, most of us subconsciously believe we will live forever. With a chronic illness or diagnosis of a terminal disease, we lose that naiveté. The fragility of life and the fact that we are here for a temporary moment in time is poignantly clear— but this recognition can become fertile ground for inner growth. Until Elizabeth Kübler-Ross published her groundbreaking book *On Death and Dying* in 1969,[20] it was not acceptable to talk about this subject with patients in a direct and straightforward way. Healthcare professionals tend to distance themselves from dying patients—perhaps from the discomfort of not knowing what to do once patients are beyond help. But this is the very time when patients need assurance that we will not abandon them in this important part of life—the process of leaving it.

WORKING WITH THE PAIN

Dr. Paul Brand devoted his life as a doctor to treating sufferers of one of the most feared and despised illnesses in human history: leprosy. His vantage point was unique; few Western doctors have experience in treating this contagious disease. Dr. Brand has lived half of his eighty years in the West, and half in India and other developing countries. I know of no other physician who has such a long track record in contrasting approaches to the medical treatment of pain across two very different societies. His experiences, recounted in the extraordinary book *Pain: The Gift Nobody Wants*, co-authored by Dr. Paul Brand and Philip Yancey,[21] help explain why some people are better able to cope with pain than others. It has less to do with physiology and individualized pain thresholds than we might think.

When Brand began his work, it had been commonly assumed that leprosy caused body parts simply to rot away—thus the characteristic facial disfigurement and loss of fingers and toes which have made lepers the object of loathing and revulsion. Brand knew, however, that the loss of body parts was rooted in the lepers' inability to feel pain in those particular body parts. Because the disease destroyed their nerve endings, they were unaware when damage was being done. Brand saw people casually reach their hands into a fire to retrieve a dropped object, or run on a broken foot, oblivious to the devastating effects on flesh and bone. Even when they were made aware of the damage and warned to take precautions, they were so desensitized by the lack of pain that they inevitably repeated the damaging behavior out of mere convenience, incurring permanent loss.

These observations fed Brand's conviction—and the central insight of his book—that "pain is no invading enemy, but a loyal messenger dispatched by my own body to alert me to some danger." Ironically, it is a gift. Ignoring or suppressing it leads to destruction. Learning to work with it reaps healing benefits.

Brand's observation of cultural differences in how people experience pain is revealing. "I was amazed by the fortitude of East Indian patients and their calm attitude toward suffering," he remarked. "Even after sitting in a crowded waiting room for hours, they did not complain. To them, pain was part of the landscape of life, and could by no means be avoided. Karma philosophy dulled any sense of unfairness about pain; it simply had to be borne." By contrast, we are obsessed with limiting pain. Unless we are aware of and on guard against this obsession, we lose the kinds of coping skills so strikingly evident among Brand's patients.

Our comfortable, materialistic lifestyle in the United States has led us to believe that we have the right and the power to avoid hardship. We feel entitled to the good life, and we feel betrayed when it is denied us. "The average Indian villager," comments Brand, "knows suffering well, expects it, and accepts it as an unavoidable challenge of life. In a remarkable way the people of India have learned to control pain at the level of the mind and spirit, and have developed endurance that we in the West find hard to understand. Westerners, in contrast, tend to view suffering as an injustice or failure, an infringement on their guaranteed right to happiness."[24]

We see pain not as a messenger, but as an enemy to be feared and avoided at all costs. Americans, who represent 6 percent of the world's population, consume 67 percent of its manufactured drugs. Yet there is little evidence that Americans feel better equipped to cope with pain and suffering. In India, according to Brand, society "has no illusions about controlling discomfort: In a country where the climate is harsh, tropical diseases abound, and natural disasters roll in with each typhoon, no one can pretend to 'solve' pain. Nonetheless, over the centuries, the culture has discovered ways to help its people cope. A society that lacked many physical resources was forced to turn to mental and spiritual resources."[25] Rather than trying to solve pain by eliminating it with technology and drugs, we would do well to listen to it and then search for the most effective ways to manage it.

Human suffering consists of outer conditions (the painful stimuli) and inner responses, which take place in the mind. Although we cannot always control the outer conditions, we can learn ways to control our inner responses. Cultures in the developing world may lack modern analgesics, but their traditional belief systems, family structures, and community support help them cope with pain. We in the "civilized" West try to manipulate our world, but natural disasters show us that we lack control and that our manipulation is often counterproductive. The same is true of our frantic attempts to control pain and manipulate the environmental and physiological factors that give rise to it. Despite our success in limiting suffering, the intensity of our drive often produces counterproductive results in coping with pain.

The ability to accept misfortune with peace of mind is a testimony to the spiritual capacity of humankind. Pastor and philosophy professor Diogenes Allen describes our common tendency to respond to suffering egotistically, with indignation and self-pity—"why did this happen to *me*?" If we allow this initial response to lead us into genuine reflection, we encounter the hard reality that we are physical beings, part of the natural order and therefore vulnerable to injury, illness, and decay. Although this recognition is humbling, it also points to the realization that we are more than *just* physical beings. We can transcend our material limitations—and in this sense, we have a spiritual dimension. This dimension is what gives us the ability to rise above "the psyche's self-serving mechanism" in responding to difficulty: "When the flow of our self-regard is painfully interrupted...reflection can lead to a new awareness of our limitations, and it may even lead to our acceptance of such limitations."

We all have opportunities to experience both sides of adversity—closing down or opening up. One choice leads to a narrow existence, dominated by stress; the other leads to a life of greater significance—an existence centered beyond the struggle. The crux of this choice, I believe, lies in the realm of the spirit.

Pain catapults us into the realm of the spiritual by forcing us to re-evaluate questions of meaning and purpose. What is all our striving for, if it leads to loss and bitter disappointment? Why do some people suffer from illness and injury while others enjoy good health and full mobility? Asking these questions will not necessarily lead to definitive answers. But they will lead us to a decision point that demands an answer from us: whether to remain trapped in negativity or to choose to move beyond the pain.

STEPS FOR THE PATH:
SEPARATING EMOTIONS FROM RAW PHYSICAL PAIN

1. *Today, I would rate my general pain level as:*

    0   1   2   3   4   5   6   7   8   9   10
    pain free   excruciating pain

2. *Reflect on how your family responded negatively to their pain and suffering. Check all that apply:*

    ☐ Responded to their pain by becoming inactive and withdrawn.

    ☐ Tended toward hand-wringing and doomsday thinking about the future, focusing only on the worst that could happen.

    ☐ Invested energy in pointing blame instead of taking personal responsibility to do something positive about their circumstances.

    ☐ Medicated their pain with drugs, alcohol, or self-destructive cycles of behavior, intensifying their suffering.

    ☐ Allowed their obsession with pain to erode their relationships and increase their isolation from family, friends, and social circles.

    ☐ Viewed religious and/or spiritual influences in their life only as triggers for guilt and shame or sources of disillusionment and hypocrisy.

3. *Reflect on how your family responded positively to pain and suffering. Check all that apply:*

    ☐ Engaged in activities that distracted them from pain.

☐ Remained positive and hopeful about the future, viewing present struggles as opportunities for personal or spiritual growth.

☐ Exhibited self-reliance instead of dependency in creating positive ways of responding to their suffering.

☐ Pursued alternative approaches to alleviating pain instead of looking for a magic formula in the next new drug or technique, easing their suffering.

☐ Reached out to others in spite of their pain, drawing inspiration and hope from their relationships with family and friends and stimulation from social interaction.

☐ Integrated religious convictions or spiritual practices as sources of meaning and purpose, giving them a larger framework for understanding suffering.

Other: _____

_____

_____

_____

4. *Suffering is the emotional response to a physiological problem. Once we recognize that we have the power to choose our responses, we can change the nature of our suffering. Reflect on how your family, cultural, or religious background has affected your present responses to pain.*

CHAPTER FOUR

THE THREE DIMENSIONS OF PAIN RELIEF

The reductive, mechanistic view of the body grants no privilege to the "integrated whole." Modern medical science has evolved for most of this century as if the mind played no part in disease…even now, the mind is seen mostly as a kind of nuisance that can cause a placebo effect that has to be factored out of studies before the "real" impact of a drug or surgical technique can be determined.

—CHIP BROWN[27]

THE REMARKABLE STRIDES in mind-body understanding, complementary medicine, and holistic approaches to health have addressed the intersection of physiology and technology with psychology and spirituality. Materialistic, Western pragmatism has been tempered by Eastern mysticism. But this integration has yet to take root in the professional healthcare community in a significant way, especially in the pain specialty. Ironically, the treatment of pain is perhaps the area most in need of such multi-dimensional understanding.

When we presume that spiritual issues are relevant only for the religiously inclined, we marginalize a central aspect of what happens in the pain experience. Perhaps the failure to acknowledge the reality of the human spirit lies at the heart of what is missing in conventional medicine. In years to come, the specialty of pain medicine may well be the branch of medical science that reintroduces this fundamental reality to our understanding of how to treat illness and alleviate suffering. But right now we are in its infant years, far behind other cultures in affirming the mysterious yet harmonious unity of the whole person. Our greatest strides in the next phase of medical science may well lie in discovering how crucial a role the human spirit plays in the healing of the whole person.

Advances in our understanding of the physiology of pain lend credence to the gathering evidence of the influence of spirit and mind on the body. It is far beyond the scope of this book to attempt a comprehensive overview of the physiology of pain. Rather, I want to broaden our understanding of how mind and body interact to show that our physiological experience of pain is a changing process rather than a static state. It is not set in stone. Fluid in nature, it is better characterized by the word "plasticity." This helps explain why certain kinds of pain often dismissed as "all in the mind" are in fact literal realities. It also affirms that pain patterns are not absolute, predetermined conditions: they are shaped not only by the kind of injury sustained, but also by an array of contributing factors. They can be intensified or modulated by an individual's responses to the pain.

Recent studies have established that prayer and meditation change the individual's response to pain. As I hope to suggest in exploring specific patterns in the physiology of pain, the interplay of the three dimensions of body, mind, and spirit is reality, not speculation. Our scientific understanding seems to be bringing us to the very boundaries of where body, mind, and spirit converge.

In its most elemental form, pain is the body's acknowledgment that injury has occurred. In this respect, all of us share a common recognition of pain. There are crucial differences, however, in how we experience pain as the message of injury is transmitted and interpreted. The best way to understand these differences lies in five key concepts: pain behavior, central sensitization, neurosignatures, the rebound trap, and brain plasticity.

PAIN BEHAVIOR

Most of us are familiar with the pain of acute sunburn. The pain signal is transmitted from the surface of the skin to the spinal cord, where it synapses (connects) with other nerves that transmit messages to the brain. Although the origin of the injury is the same from person to person, each individual recognizes the pain of the sunburn uniquely. This is due in part to physiological differences: one man's pathway will differ from another's simply because all aspects of his anatomy and physiology are unique to him and help define his individual identity. But differences in response to the injury may vary even more from one person to another because of the vastly different ways in which each of us responds to painful stimuli. You may shrug off a sunburn as a slight inconvenience while somebody else is consumed with its stinging pain and walks around stiffly for several days exclaiming, "Don't touch me!" These differing responses are varieties of pain behavior.

The nervous system transmits the message of tissue injury to the brain. Differences in pain behavior emerge from the many different ways in which this perception is either downplayed or exaggerated. Some of these variables are traceable to psychosocial backgrounds. Your unwritten family rules may have instilled the belief that pain behavior is a shameful display of weakness. Somebody else's family may foster such outward displays as a way of regulating dynamics between family members. The greatest variables in how we respond to pain lie in the emotional and spiritual realm of suffering. In the crescendoing chain of events along the spectrum of pain, suffering is by far the most individualized response. We will look more closely at that dimension in later chapters, particularly chapter five, but first it is crucial to understand how the physiology of pain determines crucial differences in our responses.

The first step in the physical recognition of injury occurs at receptor sites (specialized cells that recognize injury) all over the body. When stimulated, the receptors send messages to the spinal cord, which will then transmit them to the brain (see fig. 4.1). Once the brain receives these messages of pain, it will send reply messages back through the spinal cord and out to the peripheral site of injury.

The central nervous system functions like a vast communications system, a comprehensive network connecting all parts of the organism with the brain. Incoming and outgoing pain messages are coordinated through a region of the spinal cord called the dorsal horn (see fig. 4.2). The dorsal horn is a virtual corridor extending the length of the spinal cord, containing a "chemical soup" comprising receptors, synapses (connections between two nerve fibers), and chemical transmitters. It functions like a central railroad station between the body's superficial receptors and nerves and the headquarters of the brain. Depending on where in the body the injury occurs, the entry zone for the pain message into the dorsal horn occurs at a different point along the spine. If the injury occurred in the hands, for example, the pain message will enter the dorsal horn up in the cervical zone (neck areas) of the spine. When the feet are injured, the entry zone is the lower or mid back. This entry point serves as a kind of switching station, as the superficial nerves connect with the central nerves carrying messages directly to the brain.

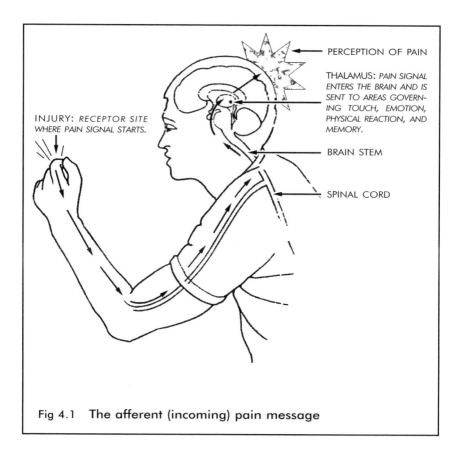

Fig 4.1   The afferent (incoming) pain message

Messages flow two ways through the dorsal horn: bottom up, from the receptor sites to the brain; and top down, from the brain to the site of injury. Within the dorsal horn, these stimuli are modified and changed. Neurotransmitters (chemicals—such as epinephrine, norepinephrine, and serotonin—that transfer messages) form a chemical soup that can either intensify or diminish the pain signal. When the alarm is sounded that injury has occurred and the pain message races up to the brain, the brain will send messages back out to the dorsal horn to modify the incoming pain signals. There may be a dampening effect on the body's alarm over the injury as the brain's way of "down-regulating" the pain pathways—in contrast to a possible "up-regulating" from the injury site to the brain, intensifying the effect.

Neurotransmitters affect both the up-regulating and the down-regulating of pain pathways. We know that pain inhibitors—not just drugs, but a life-giving relationship, a workout that stimulates endorphins, or listening to soothing music—stimulate the pathways that modulate pain. The power of positive thinking and prayer on healing has been established clinically in numerous studies. "We always knew it helped; now we have the proof," people of faith have been commenting as the research has been publicized. But now we know the scientific basis for such behavioral techniques as hypnosis, biofeedback, and relaxation exercises—even prayer and meditation. Through our understanding of how neurotransmitters regulate pain messages in the dorsal horn, we are identifying the physiology of mind-body connections.

We are not as clear yet on the physiology of how depression, anxiety, and fear intensify pain. Perhaps they somehow rearrange the ingredients of the dorsal horn's chemical soup, preventing the pain-inhibiting pathways from being activated. We do know that they are pain intensifiers.

Chronic pain patients experience repetitive stimuli from pain fibers, heightening the sensitivity of the receptors to the same stimuli. When the stimuli occur over and over again, they create an "imprint" of the pain message on the central nervous system. With acute pain, the pain message is established by the superficial nerves and eventually carried through the central nervous system to the brain, but it may be changed en route at the dorsal horn of the spinal cord. With chronic pain, the same pain message repeated continually may create an imprint that is maintained by the central nervous system long after the original painful stimulus has stopped or markedly decreased—a phenomenon known as "central sensitization." Repetitive alteration of the chemical soup of neurotransmitters and receptor-stimulators changes the way the central nervous system handles pain messages.

This mechanism for persistently repeated pain is similar to what people suffer in so-called phantom limb syndrome—they continue to feel pain in an arm or a leg that is no longer there. Phantom limb is a good model for understanding the physiology of chronic pain: the message is not imagined, because it is actually imprinted on the brain. The nervous system is still interpreting an incoming (afferent) barrage of impulses—bottom-up messages from the periphery to the center. By contrast, outgoing messages (efferent) are a top-down array of impulses carried from the central nervous system back out to the peripheries. Thus the cliché "it's all in your head" is literally true, when the phenomenon of central sensitization and imprinting have occurred. To the brain, the pain is all too real.

CENTRAL SENSITIZATION

When a traumatic event happens, it triggers a barrage of painful impulses. Repetitive incoming signals increase the intensity and frequency of the pain message in the "wind-up phenomenon," sometimes leading to an imprint on the brain. This is the process of central sensitization. The nervous system retains a physiological memory of the damage it has sustained, even if the pain impulse has been withdrawn.

THAT'S THE BAD NEWS

The good news is that understanding this physiological condition teaches us that we have control. For example, those who suffer from the disease of Raynaud's Syndrome, in which the hands are painfully cold, can learn through biofeedback to raise the temperature of their hands. They can learn to control vasodilation (expansion of the blood vessels) and constriction through therapy affecting their modulatory pathways and neurotransmitters.

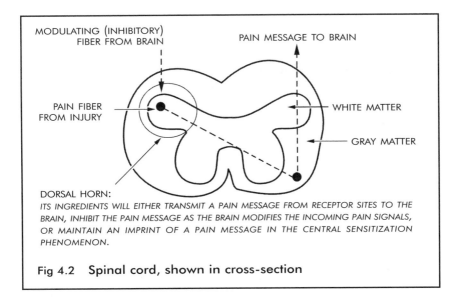

MODULATING (INHIBITORY)
FIBER FROM BRAIN

PAIN MESSAGE TO BRAIN

PAIN FIBER
FROM INJURY

WHITE MATTER

GRAY MATTER

DORSAL HORN:
ITS INGREDIENTS WILL EITHER TRANSMIT A PAIN MESSAGE FROM RECEPTOR SITES TO THE BRAIN, INHIBIT THE PAIN MESSAGE AS THE BRAIN MODIFIES THE INCOMING PAIN SIGNALS, OR MAINTAIN AN IMPRINT OF A PAIN MESSAGE IN THE CENTRAL SENSITIZATION PHENOMENON.

Fig 4.2   Spinal cord, shown in cross-section

An example of how we can benefit from understanding central sensitization is operations involving amputations. Sound research exists demonstrating that when the extremity of painful sensation is anesthetized (such as with a spinal or epidural block) before the amputation, it may markedly decrease the amount of phantom limb pain the patient eventually experiences. This is because the incoming barrage of pain signals, sent from the periphery to the central nervous system, has been blocked. Therefore, the central sensitization that might otherwise have developed, creating a blueprint of the event in the patient's brain, is markedly decreased or even eliminated. The central nervous system never receives the original message from the periphery; the wind-up phenomenon is defused before it develops; and the imprint is not allowed to form. Otherwise, without the anesthetic block, the patient's body might continue to perceive the painful injury of amputation for years to come.

Those who have had an amputation and now suffer from phantom limb pain can stimulate the inhibitory pathways through cognitive skills such as hypnosis or invoking spiritual practices to decrease the body's perception of pain.

When stimuli from our brain move down the central nervous system through the dorsal horn of the spinal cord, the perception of pain from the body's periphery can be changed. Biofeedback, hypnosis, relaxation exercises, meditative responses, and prayer come top-down from the brain to the central nervous system and can inhibit pain at the dorsal horn of the spinal cord. Instead of winding up, the pain winds down. This is a relatively simple concept, yet it is not widely known. It provides the scientific explanation for the positive effects of cognitive therapy and spiritual practices.

The wind-up phenomenon explains why people who continue to suffer from chronic pain are not just mired in a negative body-mind dynamic. They may also be experiencing pain via central sensitization. The science of neurophysiology (the study of how the nervous system functions in carrying messages from the periphery to the brain and back again) is beginning to identify specific areas of the brain and the spinal cord that are stimulated by positive, rhythmical, or repetitive thoughts. Inhibitory pathways and neurotransmitters that modulate or decrease the perception of pain have been identified in the dorsal horn of the spinal cord and other parts of the brain. It has also become clear that in parts of the nervous system, there is the capacity for change, stimulated by prayer and cognitive therapies.

When our thoughts and desires wander far away from our spiritual beliefs, medical problems become more dominant and oppressive. Health problems seem to cause less anxiety and fear if we do not feel alone with our pain. Without a spiritual context for providing an awareness of transcendence, it is all too easy for individuals to feel stuck in their pain, isolated from everything and everyone, and focused only on the reality of the pain. When they feel the freedom to turn the pain over to a source greater than themselves, they inevitably find some relief from the oppressive weight of constant suffering. This is not just an emotional response; physiologically, prayer stimulates inhibitory nerve fibers that effectively turn down the volume of pain.

NEUROSIGNATURES

Pain behavior and central sensitization are two important concepts for understanding how we experience pain. A third is "neurosignature," which refers to a particular pattern of nerve pathways unique to each individual. These recurring and highly individualized pathways are formed by our early life experiences, our attitudes, and our beliefs. In a self-perpetuating way, our neurosignature influences our emotions and behavior. It may be a blueprint for illness or wellness, for weakness or strength, for headaches and nausea, or for curiosity and pleasure.

Our neurosignature can either downgrade or upgrade painful impulses coming in from the periphery, depending in part on the nature of our pathways as they have developed over time. Like a bad habit, or conversely like a good habit, recurring impulses from the brain, along with their corresponding emotions, engage our brain's previously used nerve pathways to instruct the body. This is how our thoughts become self-fulfilling prophecies. When we are flexible enough to change our minds, we do a great deal to improve our health. Our bodies and minds are a composite of genetic predisposition and experiential adaptation. Nature versus nurture, predestination versus free will—all commingle in the unique wiring of our brains that enables us to contemplate our bodies and our existence.

Perhaps the best way to handle pain includes blending sound medical techniques with appropriate spiritual and psychological intervention. The process of applying anesthesia to a body part before the intrusion of a painful stimulus is called preemptive analgesia (to preempt the pain). This procedure is useful across many medical disciplines, including the treatment of pain patients. Otherwise, if preemptive treatment is not possible, the repeated pain message may create an imprint. Once this damage has occurred, the focus must then shift from preventing to inhibiting the pain.

THE REBOUND TRAP

The rebound trap occurs when the very medication or treatment designed to alleviate pain ironically causes it to recur. We refer to this as a biphasic response—the medicine goes out to help, but then it loops back to entrench the patient in further pain. This pattern occurs most frequently with headache pain.

For example, taking too much cafergot or narcotics or even non-steroidal anti-inflammatories can lock patients into a continual headache pattern. The medication itself becomes part of the reason for the headache in a reverberating cycle, not unlike an itch from an insect bite. The more you scratch it, because it feels so good to do so, the more you irritate the skin. In place of the original itch you have now created a new pain, which may escalate in intensity beyond the original problem.

Rebound headaches can be worse than the original headache the medication was designed to eliminate, because the treatment resets the receptor sites in the brain and becomes part of the problem instead of providing the solution. We are not sure why this happens, but we think it has to do with the saturation of the receptor sites. In order to break out of the rebound trap, the patient needs help withdrawing from the medication so that the receptor sites can be desaturated. The result will usually be an ultimate decrease in pain. Once the medication is discontinued long enough for the receptor sites to reset, it may again be helpful if appropriately reintroduced. Sometimes it is necessary to help individuals discontinue use of the medication entirely. If this does not provide a physiological solution, it may help them ease their intense focus on managing the pain and turn instead to a growing confidence in the mystery of healing.

The rebound phenomenon may be expanded beyond pharmacology more broadly to a body-mind interaction. When patients give all their attention to the pain and worry compulsively about all its varied manifestations, they get bogged down in reverberating thought patterns that simply make the pain worse. In their earnest attempt to understand their pain, their focus becomes entirely somatic (of the body). This constant preoccupation intensifies their pain. Like the pharmacological rebound, the receptors may be reset, increasing the pain, plunging the sufferer further into anxiety and perpetuating the vicious cycle.

Contrast this pain-centered focus with the responses of those in less technologically advanced cultures. I have seen Navajo women with congenital hip problems working just as hard as other women with healthy joints. Cultures that are more grounded in the natural rhythms of everyday life do not share our view of a direct association between pain and impairment. In our society, we are accustomed to popping pills

at the onset of a bodily ache because we expect the instantaneous gratification of relief. We are ill-prepared for learning how to take our limitations along with us to the job or learning to turn our focus away from the
pain toward a positive direction. The renowned behavioral psychologist
Dr. Wilbert Fordyce observed that if you have something better to do,
you hurt less.[28]

At the heart of the rebound trap is a paradox: the very thing you think is
helping you is hurting you. If you are desperate for relief, you will
naturally clutch at whatever you think is going to make the pain go away.
If the results are slow in coming, you are likely to grab all the harder—
taking three pills instead of one, escalating your conviction that
something has to be done *now*, and intensifying your distress signals to
everyone around you. Your very attempts to get help may pitch you
deeper into a spiral of despair and more pain. Lifeguards know that a
panicked person in the water, flailing around for the nearest thing to
keep him above the surface, is likely to put a choke-hold around the
neck of his would-be protector and take them both down. This is an
extreme example, but it graphically illustrates what happens when
desperation shuts out all other perspectives on reality and turns counter-
productive.

Despair and fatigue often blind us to the truth that reality is larger than
our immediate framework. Pain tends to narrow our perspective, making
it harder for us to look beyond the confines of our struggle. Even the
intense desire to conquer the pain can be a form of rebound, because it
so easily leads to a negative preoccupation.

If you are obsessed with resolving a problem, finding a way to release
your preoccupation can break your reverberating mental cycle. Let's say
you leave the office with your mind racing again and again over the
same issue. You begin driving home and realize that you can't
remember pulling out of the parking lot because your mind has been so
preoccupied. *I've got to stop thinking about this for a while, you tell
yourself, because it's getting me nowhere and if I'm not more careful I'll
end up in an accident because of it.* You turn on some music and two
miles later, while you're sitting at a red light, a solution to the problem
suddenly pops into your mind. You have just experienced breaking out
of the rebound trap.

Athletes know that there is an optimum intensity beyond which it is counter-productive, or even destructive, to push their bodies. Intuitively, they know when they reach this level. Pain patients often have this intuitive knowledge as well, but they need help in stepping back to recognize that level and refocus their attention. Once they learn how to act on this awareness, they can reverse the escalating intensity of their suffering.

Physiologically, we know that receptor sites are saturated with neuro-transmitters, and we can begin to reset them by something as simple as taking a deep breath. Many religious traditions prescribe spiritual practices that in one way or another involve breathing or meditating exercises that calm body and mind. Now we understand why these practices are so effective in breaking the cycle of pain and anxiety: they have a direct effect on how the body responds to stimuli. In the Christian tradition of the Lord's Prayer, the petition "Thy will be done" is essentially a letting go of the world's evils, turning them over to a higher source. Appropriating this prayer by taking a deep breath, sitting back from the pain, and turning it over to a transcendent power is a form of reversing the rebound cycle.

Breaking the rebound trap, however, cannot be reduced to the level of mind-body science. Although we know that receptor sites play a critical role in escalating or de-escalating pain, there is much we don't know about the body's healing power. The rebound concept plunges us into psychological and spiritual mysteries, which warrant our respect even as we strive to identify and understand them.

BRAIN PLASTICITY

One of the physiological reasons why we are able to break out of the rebound trap is the concept of brain plasticity: the ability of the central nervous system to change the way it operates. Remarkably, the body has built-in power to reverse its own self-destructive patterns and make the physiological changes necessary to move toward healing.

It is amazing to discover just how malleable the brain and the nervous system are. Much like a computer, the brain has hardware and software.

We appear to be hard-wired for certain neurologic responses. For example, stimulating the brain in a particular zone (the emetic) causes nausea and vomiting. Researchers have identified specific zones in the brain that, when stimulated by practices such as contemplative prayer and meditation, produce a sense of spiritual transcendence and awe.

But we are also soft-wired for certain things, enabling us to learn new skills and adapt thought and behavior accordingly, such as changing our ways of responding to stress with hypnosis or relaxation techniques. Brain plasticity empowers us to benefit from positive expectations. The brain is a living, changing member of our organic self. Cognitive therapy, spiritual awareness, remembered wellness, and intuitive thoughts can literally change our minds.

Herbert Benson introduced the term "remembered wellness" to replace the term "placebo effect."[29] The placebo effect tends to have negative connotations, such as the arbitrary dismissal of some recurring problems as being "all in your head." Remembered wellness is a powerful, positive term describing how we want to feel. It is rooted in our strong, natural desire for health and wholeness. "All of us project our intense desire for wellness onto the medicine we take," Benson observes. "Remembered wellness isn't particularly mysterious."[30]

Armond Trousseau, a nineteenth century French physician, advised his contemporaries to treat as many patients as possible with new drugs while the drugs still had the power to heal. Expectations of health are powerful—witness the surge of interest in herbal remedies such as melatonin and St. John's wort. Once word got around, people ran out to the store and found that melatonin helped them sleep better and St. John's wort eased their depression. To some degree, these effective results are rooted in the power of remembered wellness.

In the era when the polio vaccine and penicillin were new, we thought the power to stamp out disease was in the palm of our hands. However, epidemics such as AIDS and the increasing incidence of breast and prostate cancers humble us in the realization that we do not have the power we presumed. They return us to a more holistic, less technique-oriented way of exploring our vulnerability to disease and searching for resources with which to fight it. Technological advances have wrought wonders, but they have also tended to narrow our focus to discrete parts of the human body. We study the minute details of individual trees in disregard of their place in the forest. In our legitimate quest for the advance of medical science, we forget that until a hundred years ago the placebo effect, spiritual beliefs, and remembered wellness were the treatments of choice.

THREE-DIMENSIONAL PAIN MANAGEMENT

Because studies of the brain are yielding new evidence of how the mind controls and affects the body, the mind-body loop is easier to understand and accept. But the existence of the spirit is scientifically debatable. The spirit-body loop is observable in its manifestations: a peace that surpasses comprehension; joy in the midst of suffering and sorrow; the vital spark evident in a person whose body is rapidly deteriorating; the strong sense of a person's presence continuing after she has died; the sudden and sometimes overwhelming transformation of personality when nothing external has changed; the movement away from bitterness and anger toward forgiveness and love. When I watch the miracle of relinquishment, of turning over helplessness to trust, I witness the miracle of the human spirit coming alive.

The beauty of spirit is that we can't get our hands around it to document it. If we could, we would be all over it. How freeing it is simply to yield to its mystery in recognition that we are not able to control it. For healthcare providers and for family and close friends, there is relief in knowing that at a certain point you have done everything you can, and any further healing will be accomplished only by the mysterious power of the spirit.

Scientific advances in our understanding of how mind and body interrelate have perhaps inadvertently reduced our view of pain to a two-dimensional reality: the body experiences it, and the mind perceives it. Then a paradigm shift occurred: if you can change how the mind perceives it, then you can change how the body experiences it. This reversal is true. The body's responses to painful stimuli can be intensified or moderated by thought patterns, as cognitive therapies for pain treatment attest.

Entrenchment in chronic pain, however, can drain off energy and initiative to such a degree that nothing short of wholesale reactivation will reverse the downward spiral and turn the individual toward healing. Accomplishing this reversal requires far more than boosting willpower and adopting positive thinking. It necessitates a transformation from within. I am convinced that this inner work takes place in the realm of the spirit.

"Man lives in three dimensions: the somatic, the mental, and the spiritual," declared Dr. Viktor Frankl, a therapist who endured the catastrophic suffering of the Holocaust. "The spiritual dimension cannot be ignored, for it is what makes us human."[32] Regardless of religious convictions, most of us would agree that at the core of the human person there is a unique essence that is not reducible to mind and body alone. Frankl's third dimension describes what we mean when we say that the "spirit" of someone lives on after death, whether in the memories of others or in some perceived form of afterlife.

In the nineteenth century it was understood that what happened with the bedside doctor included care for the human spirit as well as treatment of the body. In the last hundred years, we have witnessed a split of this care into twin disciplines for healing—physical care with the doctor and spiritual care with the priest. Care of the whole person was further segmented into a third discipline, psychological dynamics, in the so-called therapeutic age. Until the very recent trend toward holistic medicine, conventional disciplines have treated body, mind, and spirit separately. What used to be one river has divided into three separate streams, none of which flows in confluence with the others.

Frankl recognized that the three disciplines belonged together. To separate them was to violate the unity of the human person. His experiences in Nazi concentration camps shaped his conviction that an individual's "will to meaning" was necessary for survival and therefore an essential dimension of human existence. He arrived at this body-mind-spirit understanding not because he was trying to explain the persistence of religion, but because he had observed something critical to our survival that is irreducible to mind or body.

Fundamental to what it means to be human, Frankl declared, is the search for meaning. This will-to-meaning is not a mere symptom of a restless mind, but an absolutely vital part of existence—the distinguishing characteristic of humans in contrast to animals. Animals do not agonize over the meaning of their existence. Yet without a sense of this meaning, humans cannot survive when all else has been stripped from them. Frankl pleaded with his contemporaries not to ignore this fundamental reality by dismissing it as a religious invention superimposed onto materialistic reality.

Other researchers have studied the human person in an attempt to identify the spiritual dimension without defining it in religious terms. Daniel Helminiak, a psychotherapist and educator, describes the human mind as a "double" reality of psyche and spirit. Therefore, human beings are spiritual by nature. The whole person is not simply body and mind or body and soul, but, organism, psyche, and spirit.[33]

In the past thirty years, medicine has changed as rapidly as the computer industry. Yet patients still have the same physical problems, the same psychological and emotional needs, the same restless longings. Technological and pharmaceutical advances may have increased life spans and decreased physical pain, but they have been far less effective in diminishing patient suffering or nurturing a sense of individual worth in the context of a caring community. It is crucial that we complement our scientific and therapeutic expertise on the physiological level with corresponding attention to the effects of pain on mental, emotional, and spiritual levels.

STEPS FOR THE PATH:
OBSERVE THE INTERPLAY OF BODY-MIND-SPIRIT

1. *Today, I would rate my general pain level as:*

0	1	2	3	4	5	6	7	8	9	10
pain free										excruciating pain

2. *How do you find yourself triggering the rebound phenomenon in dealing with your pain?*

3. *Pain behavior is manifested in actions such as wincing, limping, or constant complaining. How do you notice this behavior in others?*

    How do you notice it in yourself?

4. *Brain plasticity confirms that physiological patterns are not set in stone. Pain and suffering can be changed through the interaction of mind, body, and spirit. How do techniques or practices such as relaxation, biofeedback, hypnosis, or meditative prayer affect your experience of pain?*

5. *Finding a path to improved coping involves a personalized balance of the interplay of mind, body, and spirit. What are the next few steps in your journey of integrating the three dimensions of pain relief?*

CHAPTER FIVE

HEARTACHE: THE PAIN WE NEGLECT

[Yes,] the world's pain does break our hearts, over and over and over again. but a broken heart is not a paralyzed one...hearts are broken open, not destroyed; and from an open heart's capacity to be with suffering, healing arises.

—ELIZABETH ROBERTS AND ELIAS AMIDON[34]

S EVERAL YEARS INTO my medical career, I had a life-threatening condition that transposed me from doctor to patient. The resulting experience took me well beyond traditionally Western solutions of pills and shots and surgeries, so profoundly affecting me that I changed specialties as a result. This awakening took me deeper into my own beliefs and planted in me the desire to search for and share the meaning of the universality of pain.

In 1986, while practicing in Santa Fe as an anesthesiologist and supporting a wife and three small children, I learned that I had an enlarged heart caused by a mitral valve problem. Without treatment, I could expect an early death from congestive heart failure. The doctors, who were very guarded with their prognosis, were clear that I needed major surgery to replace the valve, with the prospect of repeated heart surgeries following it. I would also be placed on the blood-thinning drug coumadin, which would decrease my chances of an active life while increasing the risks of stroke and a multiplicity of other complications. As an avid runner and skier who enjoyed outdoor recreation with my family, I faced a severely limited lifestyle.

I was not as certain as my doctors that such high-risk surgery was my only option for treatment, but they were too busy with many other patients to research alternatives for this one problem. I felt anxious and alone, with a time bomb ticking in my chest.

At that time in my life, I had a sense of spiritual reality but had not yet built up my inner life sufficiently to draw on spiritual resources for such a life-threatening crisis. I turned to a close friend who was a pastoral counselor, and I began reading more specifically about spiritual practice. With my friend's counsel, I decided on a prayer-centered approach to building up the psychological and spiritual strength I knew I would need simply to make the decision regarding treatment. I learned to practice petitionary prayer, asking for help in love and openness as I released this overwhelming problem to a Supreme Being. I started a regular practice of prayerful meditation, which has since become a lifelong habit. And I broke the barrier of self-consciousness in asking for intercessory prayer from people in my community, including those in other denominations and religious traditions.

My pastor friend and I began by bathing everything in prayer, including the prognosis. We spent time listening and asking for guidance. His intuition was that we should not be limited by the conventions of Western medicine. Together, we developed a sense of peace that there would be a therapeutic alternative to the surgical answer. He wisely suggested that I study the problem at the university medical school library nearby. I had been an anesthesiologist on an open-heart team and would at least know where to begin.

I began to experience the quiet calm and confidence that so uniquely arises from prayer. As I continually turned over my fears and uncertainties, I found that creative ideas flowed. I discovered information quickly, as if I were being guided to just the right references. Answers that were difficult to obtain on my own came to me clearly. As I received help simply because I had asked for it, I felt increasingly sure that there was a reason for this crisis. Although there were still many uncertainties on the path ahead, I had confidence that the way would eventually become clear. Ultimately, I had hope that a deeper purpose was drawing me along.

I have observed that regardless of denomination or tradition, authentic spiritual practice—far from shutting down the intellectual dimension, as some suppose—tends to enhance cognitive thinking. The pursuit of rational knowledge combined with listening for intuitive knowledge has a powerfully synergistic effect. Techniques such as meditation, hypnosis, prayer, and relaxation exercises encourage proactive engagement, in contrast to the passivity reinforced by our healthcare system.

Among the journal stacks in the university library I found an article titled "The French Correction,"[35] by a world-famous surgeon who had been performing heart-valve repairs in France. As chief cardiac surgeon of a public hospital in Paris, with few medical and legal restraints, this doctor had developed a highly artistic method of repairing the valve, rendering replacement unnecessary. Although his operation—which had not yet been conducted in the United States—had thus far proven successful, it was not easily replicated and was quite high-risk.

After locating this seminal information, I tracked down an upcoming American Heart Association convention at which this innovative surgeon's work would be presented. When I attended to learn more about the procedure, I was able to meet the surgeon's assistant personally, and with serendipitous ease, we arranged for the operation in France.

Thanks to my immersion in the medical profession, I knew more than I wanted to know about the very dangerous physical situation I was in. My growing spiritual convictions did not spare me emotional turmoil. I often felt as if I were in a black tunnel, with no guarantee that I would ever find my way out into the light of a healthy future with my loved ones.

In the days leading up to my departure for the operation, I prepared mentally and emotionally by meditating each day in the early morning. I followed an active breathing process recommended in a book on spiritual disciplines I was reading at the time.[36] Afterward I would visualize heart and soul leaving my body and slowly rising up into the dark, early-morning sky of Santa Fe, drifting through the changing colors of the clouds into the healing presence of God. Through these interludes, I came to believe that my heart was already in the process of being healed. I sensed that the problem with my physical heart was connected to deeper issues within my soul, that my journey of physical healing was also a process of inward purification.

The night before I left for Paris, Native American friends visited me from the nearby San Ildefonso Pueblo. Dora Tse-Pe and her family arrived in their pickup truck to present a gift: one of Dora's beautiful black-on-black pots that she had made from the earth as a symbolic and spiritual gift to the French surgeon halfway across the globe. My surgery was scheduled very close to the San Ildefonso feast day, and I knew that Dora's clan would be offering prayers, dancing, and conducting religious ceremonies for me. This spirit-filled medicine was a powerful support to me—and perhaps to the surgeon as well, for the operation proved successful.

I have been privileged to lead a full and healthy life since that time, but it has been a fuller and richer life than I ever had before the crisis. I now understand from intimate personal experience that healing involves the whole person—physical, psychological, and spiritual. My heart-sickness gave me a healthy respect for the literal as well as metaphorical realities of heartache.

THE ENTWINING OF PAIN AND HEARTACHE

Everybody knows what heartache feels like. Why do we avoid talking about it in the context of pain? Heartache is not merely metaphorical: it is an authentic, bodily experience, and no less real than an ache in the lower back. Yet the realm of heartache represents the greatest divergence between professional medicine and the non-professional world of self care. Bookstore shelves in the categories of popular psychology and health are filled with variations on the common theme of holistic healing and the integral unity of the human person. Pain practice, one of the newest medical specialties, has yet to catch up with this holistic emphasis. It is still concerned primarily with technique.

Our curious neglect of heartache in professional medicine may well be rooted in our neglect of the human spirit. Physiologically, we experience pain at the mind-body level. On a spiritual level, we experience pain as heartache. These realms are profoundly and inextricably connected. When the body suffers injury, the mind and body shift into gear to help repair and heal what is broken. But if mind and body are handicapped by unrelieved pain, the human spirit will be burdened as well, and a sense of meaninglessness and despair will set in. Furthermore, if the human spirit has been injured by loss or betrayal and heartache worsens without any healing, it will have adverse effects on mind and body, intensifying pain. When these inner losses are adequately addressed and healing begins, the consequent renewal of the spirit may strengthen physiological resources, modifying pain.

It is unfortunate that we tend to dance around the issue of heartache rather than confront it, because it has core potential for the greatest change as well as for the greatest distress. But it requires humility in the face of mystery: some realities are accessible through intuition rather than observation and analysis.

I remember a patient of mine who finally found the love of his life at age fifty. They married and settled into a rewarding life together. He was even happier in his work, which he attributed to his newly fulfilling life. To his great sorrow, however, within just a few years his wife was diagnosed with a brain tumor. She died only two months after the diagnosis.

Soon after that, he began experiencing chest pain. He was diagnosed with angina, and he underwent coronary artery bypass surgery. He participated in a cardiac rehabilitation program, but chest pain continued to bother him on a daily basis, despite post-op indications that he was recuperating well. He was afraid he would either die from the pain or need further surgery.

It was his rabbi who finally helped him identify the source of the continuing pressure in his chest. This man was suffering from literal heartache. Once he began to differentiate the heartache of losing his beloved wife, from the angina he no longer had, his fear gradually subsided. But there was still the problem of his heartache, for which no bypass surgery was available.

The antidote proved to be, in part, a rekindled spiritual awareness. He'd had a spiritual sensitivity in his youth but lost it in the journey through adulthood. Now, the boy had come back to visit the man, and the spiritual nurture was life-giving. Though the process was gradual and painfully slow, his heartache eventually diminished enough to allow him once again to find periods of light and joy.

A HIDDEN PAIN

Many people come to the pain center stating what they believe to be their problem. The headaches keep recurring. The back pain is causing distress in other parts of the body.

These conditions are real, and they need genuine treatment. But often they are symptoms of an underlying problem. The root cause might be alcoholism, loss of a primary relationship, or a blow to personal identity through job loss. The true problem—that is, the need that must be addressed in order to treat the pain effectively—lies not in the physical manifestations, but in the trauma of some burden they are carrying.

Pain is the result of injury. Treating it would be much easier if we could reduce it to the consequences of direct cause-and-effect events such as touching a hot stove or slamming a finger in the car door. We have made great strides in understanding different types of pain, such as neuropathic (nerve injury), somatic (tissue injury), or bone pain. We have developed sophisticated techniques for understanding and treating these conditions with surgery and medication and specialized procedures. We have discovered the benefits of adjuvant medications, which have a different primary use but serendipitously are also effective in ameliorating pain.

The pain of heartache is just as real as what you feel when you pull a pot off a hot burner without a potholder. Yet it is curiously missing from most professional literature. I have never seen a clinical description, medical or otherwise, of heartache. In our society, we tend to avoid talking about it except in rare conversations with our closest friends, or we cloak it in flippant humor. I believe we need to add it to our list of pain types.

We are a long way from understanding how to treat heartache. For the most part, it does not respond to treatment by medication. It is a mind-body experience, weighted perhaps more heavily in the mind, but definitely felt in the body. For some it is almost literally a wrenching sensation, as if the heart is being torn from the chest. Whatever its origin—the death of a loved one, the end of an intimate relationship, or the loss of a child—heartache is a very real pain that merits attention and treatment just as much as an ache in any other part of the body.

Some might prescribe the antidote to heartache as a visit to a therapist, perhaps in conjunction with medication prescribed by a psychiatrist. For a lucky few, that may be the beginning of the end to that particular heartache. But heartache is not necessarily synonymous, or even associated, with depression. For many, it must simply be endured as a daily experience until in time and by grace, the ache gradually diminishes.

Much of the time, heartache remains a hidden pain. I wonder if we tend to neglect it because our mad dash through schedules and commitments keeps us so disconnected from our inner life. The movement toward simplicity in recent years reflects our rebellion against such fragmented, outer-directed living. In years past, our forebears may have lacked the conveniences of technology, but at least they had built-in opportunities for slowing the mind and easing the spirit while riding a horse across the fields or walking to their next destination. We transport ourselves in self-enclosed bubbles equipped with tools and toys to keep us productive and preoccupied. At home, the incessant drone of television conveniently fills in the empty spaces between activities, further distancing us from the potentially healing power of solitary reflection and inner renewal.

If it doesn't catch up with us in our daily routines, heartache will inevitably visit us in the lonely night hours. If we suppress it there as well, it will likely come back to revisit us in physical and mental distress. It can be a very insistent and demanding form of pain.

A VERY REAL PAIN

Heartache is a hidden pain also because it is rooted in some of the most personal and private experiences of life. It is bound up in the inner life, and so it cannot be objectified or defined in the recognizable function of a particular body part.

Fundamentally, heartache is pain felt on the level of the spirit. It is a hurt that manifests itself in body and mind but extends well beyond. We speak of feeling heavy-hearted or light-hearted because these terms accurately describe the physical sensations. Yet these sensations are the results of intangible realities, perceived at an intuitive level. They are no less real—and are often more devastating to overall well-being—than is pain entering the body via receptor sites.

Body-mind healing exercises such as appropriate touch and meditation will certainly help alleviate heartache, because the human person is an integral unity. The growing trend in healthcare today is to treat "the whole person." This is a good and necessary development. We are more sensitive than ever before to the ways in which mind and body interrelate in coping with illness or injury. We know that we have an innate drive toward wholeness, and that the mind has great power to facilitate the body's natural desire for healing.

The increasing popularity of so-called complementary medicine, which combines traditionally Western medicine with alternative healing approaches, reflects our deepening understanding of the inextricable unity of mind and body. Yet we still tend to separate heartache from medical treatments, consigning heartache to a support level and perhaps bringing in a chaplain. To treat the whole person requires physicians to pay attention to heartache as a foundational, not a peripheral, aspect of the pain experience.

For those suffering pain from a life-threatening condition, treating the whole person includes relating proactively to loved ones and family members, if the patient is fortunate to have such support nearby.

While I was recovering from my heart operation in Paris in a hospital primarily for patients from former French colonies, I avoided special privileges such as seeking pain medication frequently. Since I was a curiosity among the patients, I was trying not to be the ugly American. I sought ways to deal with the discomfort common to all of us, so that the other patients could accept me and I could participate with them in the healing process.

After surgery, I was on a ward of nine people, most of whom were from Africa—Mauritania, Ivory Coast, Algeria, and Tunisia. Others were from Italy and Greece. None spoke the same language. Patients were cared for by their relatives, most of whom stayed with them at the hospital— nursing them, feeding them, sleeping under their beds. At first the sight of all these people startled me, but it quickly became clear that they were not intruders, and in fact quite the opposite. They came not only to help their loved ones, but others as well.

My companions included a nine-year-old with congenital heart disease who sat on my bed and drew pictures for me. I remember trying to focus attention away from pain into his eyes and onto his pictures. An "earth-motherly" Italian woman would scurry out of the hospital to get *biftec* for the American physician who looked so *blanco-blanco*. She fed me as if she were a mother bird, shoving little pieces of food into my mouth. I received massages from the family of the man from the Ivory Coast. The first time I ventured to the one bathroom on the ward, I was assisted by an Algerian patient on one side and a Tunisian patient on the other, helping me with my chest tubes and IVs. A week later, I was doing the same for the next patient coming to the ward.

In our mental, spiritual, and physical touch with one another, our ward formed a little United Nations of pain. Language and customs defined our differences, but we were united in our common trauma of heart surgery and in the compassionate caring we gave to one another.

This community of wounded individuals had more power to facilitate genuine healing than did all the pain medication dispensable through an IV within the four walls of a sterile, isolated recovery room in a state-of-the-art hospital. Each time an injured patient came out of surgery, he was immediately enveloped in an atmosphere of personal warmth.

Words were few, but communication was profound as we joined in the common task of helping everyone get better. These loving acts drew me past mental preoccupation with the pain into active participation in a community healing process. How much I would have missed had I taken a purely pharmacological approach to recovery!

My Paris experience represents yet another paradox in our society—we think it is advanced care to have a private room with the most monitors and technology, while screening out visitors and relatives. In fact, healing may be more rapid and effective when patients are surrounded by many people. Intensive care is often the most isolating. So-called advanced treatment sometimes obstructs a hands-on healing process. Ironically, what is considered the best treatment compared with the most primitive treatment actually may reverse the expected outcome.

Perhaps heartache is rarely addressed in the context of illness and pain because we tend to fragment the human person into component parts—body here in the biological sciences, mind over there in the psychological disciplines, and spirit consigned to religious traditions. The heart we leave to writers and composers. In the discipline of pain treatment, we do not have the luxury of narrowing our focus to one component part. In fact, the failure of such specialized scrutiny is often why patients are referred to us at the pain center.

The most effective starting point in treating heartache in the context of pain management may simply be to recognize it as an inevitable aspect of the pain experience. Sympathetic recognition of what others are struggling with can be a powerful facilitator in their healing.

In our medical system, the patient's passive isolation is broken only by visits from the nursing staff for impersonalized routine tasks. The only action expected of the patient, other than cooperating with these tasks or exercises to regain movement is pushing buttons for the television or for assistance. Our culture's premium on entertainment extends to the way we design our hospitals. Rather than giving people tasks for helping themselves and others, we separate them from each other and give them a television set for a companion. We rely on medication and entertainment to treat their pain. Visitors file in and out for brief exchanges—a gift of flowers, a quick squeeze of the hand, a whispered "we're praying for you." These gestures may be genuine expressions of caring, but they lack the power of sustained human presence.

The hectic pace of our routines, the demand to cluster tasks so that we are always doing two or three things simultaneously, the urgency to get where we're going faster, the drive to beat the clock and get more done in the limited time we have—all of this propels us right over the heads and hearts of suffering individuals. Rarely do we simply sit in silence, giving others the unhurried attention of compassion—the genuine desire to understand what they are going through, the attempt to feel something of what they are feeling, the assurance that their suffering is not ignored or overlooked. Genuine compassion moves beyond brief rituals of pity in seeking to ease the burden of pain in any way possible. Sometimes, entering into another's heartache is best communicated silently, through the mysterious and wordless language of the human spirit.

HEART-FELT GRIEF OVER LOSS

Most of us associate heartache with the loss of primary relationships, but it is a frequent companion to illness, especially terminal illness. When seventeenth-century British poet and cathedral dean John Donne wrote *Devotions upon Emergent Occasions*, he described with remarkable clarity of detail both the physical and spiritual implications of his life-threatening illness. In the fifth of twenty-one brief meditations chronicling the progress of his disease from onset to recovery, he described the experience of isolation:

> As sickness is the greatest misery, so the greatest misery of sickness is solitude, when the infectiousness of the disease deters them who should assist from coming; even the physician dares scarce come. ...[The] height of an infectious disease of the body is solitude, to be left alone. For this makes an infectious bed equal, nay, worse than a grave, that though in both I be equally alone, in my bed I know it and feel it, and shall not in my grave; and this too, that in my bed my soul is still in an infectious body, and shall not in my grave be so.[37]

This passage resonates with a deep awareness of loss of relationship and of bodily health. Here, Donne mourns the toll his disease has exacted on his physical well being, but also in his separation from relationships. The awareness is so painful that death would be a relief— not simply an end to suffering, but an end to his consciousness of its effects.

Pain sufferers are continually made aware of their loss of health and the multitude of other, daily losses in the simple routines and pleasures of life that are no longer accessible to them. The medical profession has made great strides in treating the physical and psychological effects of pain, but it has yet to address the effects of chronic pain upon the human spirit. Heartache reveals that to understand the complexities of the pain experience, we must move beyond the body-mind loop into the body-mind-spirit loop.

Heartache is a recognition of loss, and therefore an experience of mourning. When a marriage ends, there is mourning for the life together that was lost. When illness strikes, there is mourning for the healthy life that has vanished. Veterans of open-heart surgery will sometimes describe a curious awareness of a profound before-and-after difference: something is lost when the heart is stopped in order for the surgery to be performed; one is never again the same.

Heartache over a disruption in the body's health is a genuine inner knowing, an intuitive apprehension that is no less real simply because we cannot pinpoint its location in the body. The mind may or may not be consciously aware of the body's loss, because this kind of loss is not always perceived on a cognitive level. Nor is it simply an emotional response to a bodily event, such as an operation, which will fade with time. The knowledge of loss to the body remains.

The late writer Andre Dubus was a former Marine Corps captain, an athletic man who loved baseball and running. At age forty-nine, he stopped along a highway to help people who had just been in a car accident. He escorted a wounded woman and her brother to the side of the road and turned to flag down help from another motorist. But instead of stopping, the oncoming car swerved suddenly and plowed into them. Dubus pushed the woman out of the way. She survived; her brother died; and Dubus recovered from his injuries sufficiently to spend the rest of his life a paraplegic in a wheelchair. "After the dead are buried, and the maimed have left the hospitals and started their new lives," he wrote, the healing process starts with the "transcendent and common bond of human suffering," which eventually gives rise to forgiveness and love. In the recovery from injury, he described how "the physical pain of grief has become, with time, a permanent wound in the soul, a sorrow that will last as long as the body does."[38]

The physical organ of the heart is often used metaphorically to represent the seat of the soul, or spirit. Perhaps we should pay more attention to this. Heartache is evidence of a wound to the spirit, a disruption of our fundamental sense of self. Perhaps that is why the ache is so deep and profound. We sustain minor losses regularly—worsening eyesight, decreased muscle strength with lessened activity, fluctuations in social status and self-esteem—but they do not necessarily cause heartache. When the perception of loss is severe or deeply rooted, we grieve over the sense of having lost a part of ourselves irretrievably.

Acute or sustained pain of the body can reverberate in pain of the spirit. Conversely, when we suffer injury or illness that is not a physiological event, such as emotional wounds in the loss of a primary relationship, the associated pain can reverberate in pain of the body—headaches, depression, anxiety, stomach pain, and other physical symptoms. Because mind, body, and spirit are interconnected, no matter where pain originates it will inevitably affect the whole person if left unattended. Figure 5.1 illustrates the cyclical nature of the pain experience.

Technically speaking, we cannot experience wholeness of the body without physical health. Spiritual wholeness, however, does not require physical wholeness. The well-being of the spirit is affected but not determined by the health of the body.

Wholeness is an integration of all aspects of the human person—physical, mental, emotional, and spiritual. A high percentage of pain patients are in crisis because their relationship with their soul is weak.

When illness or injury occurs, we want a remedy that will make the problem go away completely. But that is not healing. That is a cure.

Writer Nancy Mairs (a self-described Catholic feminist) discovered this distinction one afternoon while attending Mass. In "the interior jumble that forms my post-communion meditations," she was reflecting on her rapidly worsening multiple sclerosis. She realized that her "resolve to cope bravely, in a manner befitting my stern Yankee heritage, was weakening even faster than my muscles were. I just wanted to get rid of the damned disease. 'God, God, God,' I prayed, 'please, heal me!' And then, for the first and only time in my life, I got a response...Three monosyllables simply materialized in my consciousness: 'But I am.'"

She realized that she had asked for the wrong thing. She had wanted to be cured of the disease entirely, to resume the life she used to have, to live even more fully with a healthy body. But instead she had asked for healing: "not to be freed from my limp or my nasty habits, which might be effected instantaneously, but to be made whole, which might entail collecting scattered fragments and painstakingly fitting and gluing them into place."[39]

HEARTACHE AND HEALING

While paying close attention to the recovery of the whole person, I work very hard at mending the body. Continuing professional education improves the likelihood that I will find successful ways to treat patients. For example, I attended a conference of the International Spinal Injection Society on new techniques for treating neck pain. Learning the procedure for treating cervical facet (side joints in the neck) arthritis is difficult, but it can markedly decrease certain types of headache, neck pain, and shoulder pain. After returning from the conference and practicing skills I learned there, I found I was able to help many patients who had suffered from post-whiplash injuries for years.

Of course, not everyone experiences concrete improvements. With some patients, we travel together the slow and very arduous road toward healing without immediate and dramatic improvements. For these sufferers, there is no way of taking away the scar tissue around their nerves. But I can help take away the scar tissue around their hearts.

Christian tradition refers to Christ as the "great physician." The Gospel narratives record many instances of physical healing, but Christ made it clear that miraculous cures were not the object of his ministry. They were signs of the kingdom of God, which he was ushering in. He restored wounded bodies, but he also healed broken spirits. Blessed are the heartbroken, for they shall be comforted.[40]

Many years and life experiences later, I am still experiencing the spiritual healing that has come from the crisis with my health. I am grateful that the surgery was completely successful, and I am able to live an active, normal life without medication. But truly, the heart of the matter was operated on in more than just one way. During that experience I learned

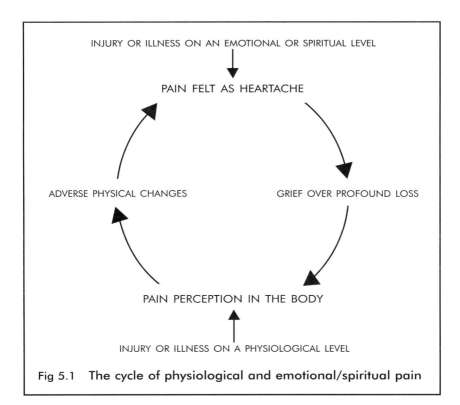

Fig 5.1   **The cycle of physiological and emotional/spiritual pain**

a profound truth that is one of the hidden blessings of pain: even in the loneliest or most painful times there is a grace in the wilderness. "The people who survived the sword found grace in the wilderness," declared the Old Testament prophet Jeremiah to the Hebrew nation.[41] Israel had been defeated by the Babylonians and taken captive in prolonged exile. From this period of defeat and destruction, the people were being offered new hope and new promise. Pain can herald a new promise of profound change, if we have eyes to see the opportunity and heart to walk through the wilderness of confusion and loss.

It is not possible to suffer the pain of a life-threatening illness, whether you are the victim or a victim's loved one, without experiencing the heartache of impending loss. Our neglect of this spiritual wound makes it much harder for us to deal with major losses. It is hard enough simply to cope with the mechanics of treating illness and its accompanying injury to the body. It is even harder, in our society, to draw upon resources for coping with the effects of illness and pain upon the human spirit.

EMBRACING MYSTERY

American society still clings to the notion that if you live right, you can avoid pain; and if you have pain, there must be something wrong with you. We are obsessed with making sense of life, with controlling pain and eradicating suffering. We demand solutions. But we seldom mention *mystery*—not a temporary ignorance that will disappear with more scientific information, but a reality essentially beyond human understanding. Appreciating the role of prayer and meditation in healing, understanding the relationship between spirituality and health, requires us to cultivate an acquaintance with mystery.

Our culture jettisoned long ago the idea that medicine and religion are the twin traditions of healing. The Medicine Man of the North American Indians embodies this concept. I saw it dramatized in the life of one of my patients, a woman whose journey took her through two very different cultures.

I met Virginia Begay when she was admitted to the University of Colorado for treatment of choriocarcinoma (retained placental parts) after the birth of her third child. If diagnosed late, this cancer has a very poor prognosis. While I was making preoperative rounds, I found Virginia receiving a unit of blood on the oncology ward. She appeared to be Native American, and I presumed that she was far away from home in a big city hospital and therefore bewildered by her surroundings. I began explaining to her in an exaggeratedly simple manner why she was receiving blood. The twinkle in her eyes as she gave me an intelligent and articulate reply exposed my error immediately, as I realized she was a well-educated woman. Instead of treating me scornfully, she gently made me aware that she understood her medical problems and the Western treatment she was receiving for them.

Virginia was fundamentally and culturally Navajo, although she was a college graduate and seemed to walk in two worlds simultaneously. She had initially gone to the Navajo "sing" man when she first got sick, but as her illness progressed she sought Western medicine as well, and began chemotherapy treatments. She firmly believed that she needed to keep one foot in the camp of her traditional Medicine Man. She wore a pouch around her neck, and she participated with her family in healing procedures. For her, Native American tradition and Western medicine were not mutually exclusive.

The Pueblo Indians of the Southwest, neighbors of the Navajos, have often thrived in two worlds simultaneously, practicing the Catholicism that was introduced to them centuries ago intermingled with their own nature beliefs. Native Americans have a very pragmatic attitude toward healing. They have no qualms about mixing various healing ceremonies. They are humble in their openness to the potential for success in other people's ways of healing. In contrast to Western culture, which presumes that theirs is the only way, Navajos easily accept the mystery that two entirely different treatments can work together to heal.

Anemic and in constant pain when I first met her, Virginia was struggling with shortness of breath and nausea induced by her medication. I remember being in her room one day when her father, a traditional Navajo wearing a great big cowboy hat, walked into the room and started speaking to her in their native tongue. Virginia relaxed into what appeared to be a hypnotic trance. As her father began chanting, peacefulness settled over the entire room. Indeed, each time family members arrived and invoked the traditional life by chanting, singing, or using power objects, there was a palpable serenity in the room.

Subsequently, Virginia's cancer metastasized to her lungs, and she was sent to a hospital in Houston to try yet another method of healing. She and her husband and their three sons became friends with my family. When I moved to Albuquerque to begin practice as an anesthesiologist, we maintained close contact.

I did not get to see Virginia again after she was transferred to Houston. As the futility of further treatments became evident, she discontinued her chemotherapy, disconnected her IVs, and with the help of her sister made the journey back home to Haystack, New Mexico. She had chosen to die in the traditional Navajo way, surrounded by friends and family. We were invited to participate in her ritual of dying, but unfortunately we received the message too late. In the high desert landscape of her youth, Virginia finally found relief from pain.

Virginia's family told us that she became calm, comfortable, and serene at the end. It often happens that people who are in excruciating pain will inexplicably have a day or two of lucidity and comfort immediately before their death. I wonder if this manifestation from deep within is a renewal of the fundamental, spiritual self.

Ultimately, what had given Virginia the ability to face her circumstances with acceptance instead of fear was not the Western science of treating disease and managing pain, but the spiritual grounding in her ethnic and tribal heritage. For Virginia, the primacy of spiritual reality was the only meaningful context for dealing with her pain and facing the consequences of her illness.

Other cultures and religious traditions have much to offer us as we cope. Their differing perspectives on illness and suffering can help us change our responses to pain in profoundly helpful ways. Recognizing heartache as injury to the spirit, and responding to it with spiritual resources, may be the first step on the path to healing and wholeness.

Somewhere in your town or city there is a child with a terminal illness. The child's relatives and friends have a deep injury to the spirit—heartache. They are praying for a miracle. The child may die right on schedule, and there still may be a miracle. It may be a renewed prayer life for the relatives. It may be the coming together of estranged family members. Or the miracle may simply be the gradual and graceful repair of the human spirit in the lessons learned from the waning heartache.

STEPS FOR THE PATH:
RECOGNIZING INJURY TO THE SPIRIT

1. *Today, I would rate my general pain level as:*

    0   1   2   3   4   5   6   7   8   9   10
    pain free   excruciating pain

2. *The word "heart" is often used metaphorically—heartbreaking news, heartfelt joy, heartwarming experiences—to point to intangible realities rather than in literal reference to the physical organ. In this chapter, heartbreak has been defined as injury to the spirit. Do you believe that injury to the spirit can intensify your physical pain?*

3. *Physicians often neglect heartache in treating pain because it is not reducible to direct observation. What hidden heartaches are you carrying that might be intensifying your physical pain?*

4. *Reflect on how nurturing your spirit has helped you recover from injury to the heart.*

CHAPTER SIX

ENERGIZING THE SPIRIT

Your soul is not a passive or a theoretical entity that occupies a space in the vicinity of your chest cavity. It is a positive, purposeful force at the core of your being.

—GARY ZUKAV[42]

S PIRITUALITY HAS COME OF AGE in recent years. What used to be embarrassingly passé is now popular. For many, religion provides a helpful way to organize life around an inner center. It keeps us from becoming mired in the superficial and materialistic. It ritualizes our need to take time out and pay attention to the intangibles, to nurture the self we often neglect in our rush to do and achieve and consume. It is not easy to take time out from schedules and demands to practice the life of the spirit. It is a gift to be compelled to do so, and that is the blessing that accompanies the curse of pain. The very thing you've been putting off, which you said you would get around to someday, has become a necessity. You are catapulted into this need to move beyond the physical plane of life not just when you get to it, but *now*: this is the place where you will find the help you need to carry the burden of illness.

As with anything trendy, spirituality can be trivialized as little more than a pleasurable experiment on the path to self-enhancement. Those in pain do not have the luxury of pursuing self-enhancement hobbies. Their need is raw and immediate. The resources they turn to must hold up under pressure that would buckle anything inauthentic.

I was once called in to manage the pain of a forty-four-year-old woman dying of adenocarcinoma of the lung, found in only about 7 percent of total lung cancer cases. Martha Conley's affluent family had been able to afford experimentation with a multitude of alternative treatment therapies. Following her lung biopsy they had pursued macrobiotic therapy in California and from there went to Mexico for even more non-traditional care. Martha's husband was a strong advocate of psychology-based approaches to defeating illnesses, especially meditation techniques and intentional thought processes. When they learned about the variety of alternative practices available in Santa Fe, he championed the family's move.

Sadly, before long Martha was admitted to the hospital emergency room in extreme pain. As soon as her husband left the room, Martha turned to the nurses and begged them for help. The nurses were able to get her admitted to our extended care wing, called El Cariño (for cariñoso, caring). When I arrived, discussions had been underway concerning pain medication. Martha was anxious, confused, and exhausted. Her husband disapproved of pharmacological methods for handling his wife's pain, but he began to relent. We started treatment with different kinds of oral narcotics, anti-emetics, and patches placed on the skin to act as long-acting narcotic reservoirs. Eventually, Martha required IV narcotics to control her pain.

When I first went in to meet Martha, I held her hand and listened to the person inside the wasting body. We talked about her pain and fear and her desire for a sense of peace. As the question arose of how to accomplish this, I felt compelled to discuss non-denominational, generalized spirituality and asked about her background. She had been raised as an Episcopalian, although she had not been in a Christian church for years. Over the years she had toyed with so-called New Age ideas, but she had jumped from one system to another with little depth or staying power.

After about three sessions Martha eventually identified that deep within her was a belief in a loving Father, in the person of Jesus who suffered for our sins. We discussed the suffering of the saints in every religion— the difficult, painful deaths of many of the apostles, of many well-known gurus in other traditions, and most assuredly the painful suffering of

Jesus on the cross. It took several sessions for her to begin developing a sense of affirmation that she was in good company if people like this could suffer. We reflected on how our lives are brief and transient moments in the span of existence. Pain brings us to our knees, giving us the opportunity to look toward eternity.

Martha's intense anxiety began to drain away as peace welled up within her. We called a local Episcopal priest, a warm and loving man who helped her deepen this peace and gain some closure. Martha had been estranged from her mother for years, but they reestablished communication across the bridge of forgiveness. Two sons also arrived. Joy and sorrow intermingled as wonderful reunion moments took place in her room in the midst of suffering. Her husband had become much more accepting of the benefits of Western medicine, and her relatives approached the reality of her impending death with a sense of peace and purpose.

This upper-middle-class woman, lulled by material comfort, had ignored her spiritual search for years. When all else fell away, the spiritual was the only realm that held any hope for her. She was able to reach deep down within to the fragments of belief and come up with the recrudescence of what was true for her. She did this in a remarkably short time, and it gave her a powerful sense of peace and *raison d'être*. Just as anxiety markedly accentuates pain, so does peacefulness markedly inhibit its intensity. The pain still afflicted her, but only intermittently, and it was overridden by her quiet confidence.

Illness and pain compel patients to find their own authentic faith. For some, this spirituality is well-defined. For others, it is a misty, uncharted landscape. We have so many choices and listen to so many different voices, it can get in the way of staying with one set of beliefs long enough to practice them. Many of us were started off as children in some kind of religious tradition that we abandoned along the way or perhaps even came to resent. Yet at least a seed was planted that could later be revitalized. I have seen how this early influence can be harvested years later to bear fruit in a spiritual awakening that yields a new sense of meaning.

Material comfort sometimes breeds the delicious illusion that we can skate comfortably along the surface of life from one pleasant destination to the next. When the ice cracked open for Martha, she had a lot of work to do. But even this eleventh-hour change opened up a larger world that gave new meaning to her life while she was preparing to leave it.

In the broadest sense, renewing the spirit means doing whatever helps you grow inwardly, to strengthen you for dealing with the physical pain. Spiritual practice is a profoundly effective way to be beyond the moment. When you're inside pain, you are trapped in the moment. When you can transcend the moment, you are moving into something bigger than the pain. Each time you acknowledge and act on whatever is spiritually authentic for you, you are building a life larger than your pain. It will not happen all at once. Just as physical exercise will help you build body strength and mental exercise will help keep your mind active, regular spiritual practice will nourish your inner life. As you keep taking steps forward in your journey of faith, the larger context in which you find meaning and purpose beyond the pain will become more real to you.

Until the fairly recent emergence of complementary medicine, conventional treatment and alternative health have been on opposite ends of the spectrum between evidence-based science and non-scientific metaphysics. Although the dichotomy is beginning to ease, there will be a need to inform physicians about your intent to seek spiritual resources while participating in concrete Western medicine. This hasn't always been the case, however.

SPIRITUALITY: A STRANGER TO THE HEALTHCARE SYSTEM

In *Prayer: The Heart's True Home*, Richard Foster observes that the distinction between priests, psychologists, and physicians is a relatively recent one.[43] In the past, the physician of the body, the physician of the mind, and the physician of the spirit were the same person. The ancient Hebrews, in particular, saw persons as a unity, and for them it would be unthinkable to minister to the body without ministering to the spirit. The *Zohar*, a thirteenth-century work of Jewish mysticism, advises the physician that if he "cannot give his patient medicine for his body, he should [at least] make sure that medicine is given him for his soul."[44]

Treating pain patients forces healthcare professionals back to an earlier era in which doctors relied on the art of medicine, rather than on the science of medicine, to facilitate healing. The doctor's responsibility is not simply to alleviate pain, but to help patients reframe an illness discussion to a wellness belief. For most patients, what is wrong with the body is far outweighed by what is right with the body. Enlisting the strength of the healthy parts will help shore up the weak parts. The dispiriting thought, "I am not well," needs to be replaced with the affirmation, "I am a well person with a problem." Physicians can encourage their patients to participate actively in their own wellness—to recognize their gifts, including their unique spiritual strengths, as powerful catalysts to the healing process.

Our culture has traditionally drawn clear boundaries between religion and science, the invisible and the visible, the intuitive and the verifiable. If it is hard for pain patients to accept the mystery of healing, it may be even harder for physicians. They are trained to raise questions in order to find answers. A healthcare provider raised on lab tests will find it difficult to shift gears into the mystery of the spiritual. But these realms are not mutually exclusive. The reality of the broken or maimed part does not mean physician and patient cannot simultaneously explore the spiritual. Physicians are slow to take the lead here, because it is not concrete. They are used to dealing with identifiable cause and effect. Once they learn to respect mystery, however, they become more mature physicians. They can celebrate the journey of healing with their patients without having to understand it. If a patient improves inexplicably, they can embrace the progress instead of obsessing over why it occurred.

Sometimes it is necessary to leave the questions unasked in order to provide what the patient truly needs at a given moment. *Why me?* is not so much a question as a cry of suffering. When patients are grappling with why they are having pain, I have been known to launch into scientific explanations of neuropathways, dorsal horn of the spinal cord physiology, and neurotransmitter linguistics. If I notice that patient and relatives grow distracted and their eyes glaze over, I will ask solicitously, "Would you like me to explain that again?" "No, that's quite all right, doctor," they inevitably reply.

There is a time for consolation, not explanation. When your best friend agonizes, "What did I do to deserve this?" you don't chronicle her personal weaknesses, trying to identify causal factors. You reassure her of your commitment to be there for her. Sometimes, what patients need most from doctors is simply a few minutes of human presence to buffer the delivery of information.

Americans spend billions of dollars each year on alternative therapies, in part because the traditional doctor-patient relationship has deteriorated. Alternative medicine more often meets the patient's need for a hands-on relationship rather than an impersonal transaction. It often does so with appropriate touch, something that technology-based care has insidiously abdicated. Physicians are far more effective when they not only care *for* patients but also *about* them. When people are sick, their functioning is reduced to a level akin to that of children and animals. They survive on intuition and instinct, and they can usually sense the other person's true level of interest or concern. Faith in the physician can help facilitate healing; distrust or feeling depersonalized can help thwart healing.

Most pain patients have already been failed by the promise of more sophisticated technology or a more efficient healthcare system. They need a doctor who will look at the whole person before assessing what is best for the hurting parts. Perhaps more than in any other area of conventional medicine, pain management is dependent upon the model of partnership between physician and patient. The hierarchical model, in which the patient passively submits to the authority of a professional who dictates treatment like a military superior assigning orders, simply does not work. The partnership model requires many changes in the way we currently practice medicine. For patients, it means an open exchange of information and insight, a willingness to learn and to put into practice the mind-body techniques that can alleviate the pain.

In the evolving world of managed care, sometimes called "care of the managers," I find myself in frenetic, chaotic, and time-squeezed circumstances. In addition to my work at the pain center, I am often called into surgery to perform as an anesthesiologist. Many years ago, anesthesiologists made preoperative visits. They got to know the patient, explained the surgical procedure, and addressed some of the pain from the anxiety and fear at the eleventh hour before surgery. Now, it is increasingly difficult to focus on patients' pain and anxiety. Many patients are admitted and released on the same day of surgery, and they see me for only a few minutes before their procedure.

In the past I would have held the patient's hand or taken the patient's pulse, sat down by the bedside, and listened. In this encounter, I would develop a sense of the patient as a person, beyond just the raw medical condition. We would discuss the operation. During the physical exam, I would thoroughly listen to the heart and lungs and examine the airway and appropriate anatomy, all the while attempting to be reassuring. This encounter with the patient took time.

Now, in the managed care system, I have less than two minutes to do a history, perform a physical, and project an authentic concern for the patient. Then, off we go to surgery. I usually give something intravenous to alleviate fear and anxiety. I catch myself saying the same thing to each patient. There is a sense of hurry I am sure the patients pick up. Some of them want to get this over with and move on, but most would like genuine interest and expertise from the anesthesiologist. Because of the speed at which the operation must be performed, all the professionals involved—the scrub nurse, the circulating nurse, the recovery nurse, the surgeon, and the anesthesiologist—develop what I call a "mode of automaticity."

In the moments right before an operation, I no longer have time to watch for cues, whether spiritual or psychological, for how a particular patient is approaching this intervention. If the patient wants prayer from a spouse or minister, it is almost impossible for me to notice it. In the past, as the patient was going to sleep, I would have tried to affirm or reinforce the spiritual beliefs manifested by the patient or by the family.

Healthcare workers will often intone, "Just relax," as if this were possible for someone who has spent a lifetime being anxious over intervention. This one-size-fits-all approach overlooks how complicated and individualized the pain experience is. The patient's perceptions of pain may be rooted in their belief systems, woven into their expectations, and intensified by fears from childhood. Pharmacology may or may not alleviate pain, but using it as the exclusive treatment ignores other pain generators—anxiety, fear, and loneliness.

In this day of less hands-on attention and more hands-off mechanisms, pain management centers become almost the first line of defense with many patients. It may be here that the patient is touched and fully examined for the first time. The pain center is the natural place to listen for clues of spirituality and the natural place for complementary medicine. This is often the first place where the patient is touched appropriately—physically, psychologically, or spiritually—by medical care professionals.

Our pain center blends left-brain and right-brain approaches—the search for concrete, empirically verifiable interventions as well as the Native American way of embracing mystery and seeking harmony. Since we are open to many alternatives, we can avoid the therapeutic tunnel vision of simply writing prescriptions or doing procedures. We are often fortunate to see direct results of specific interventions, but we don't have to attribute overall success to a specific modality alone. We respect the reality of our patients' suffering, honor their journey through it, and celebrate the mystery of healing in its many forms without demanding solutions.

When we learned that one of our patients was dealing with the death of his daughter, we called him as soon as we heard about it. The next time I saw him, I simply put my arms around him. As I felt his tears on my shoulder, I wondered if he had ever been hugged by another man. This man had endured many procedures when he came to us, most of them unsuccessful. We were able to modulate the pain with some appropriate adjuvant non-narcotic medication, but our greatest help, I think, has been a strengthening from within. He is a different person, emotionally and spiritually, than the man who first walked through our doors. He was catapulted into a dimension of life he had never known before, and he now has a strong sense of his own inner growth. He feels a certain accountability to us for this new development, and he no longer goes to a primary-care physician. He comes to the pain center twice a month not so much for the back pain, but because we're the only ones who have recognized that his grief is more significant than the pain from his back surgery.

Although physicians readily make referrals for psychological support or physical therapy, most tend to be uncomfortable with helping patients get spiritual support consistent with their patient's religious background or current beliefs. Many of them are now recognizing, however, that this factor has as much potential as any other aspect of medical care to meet patients' needs—not by taking the place of those other approaches, but by complementing them in laying a foundation of support for the healing process. Some healthcare workers may feel it is intrusive to listen for cues to a patient's spiritual beliefs, but more and more patients are asking to be treated as a whole person, including the request for spiritual support in times when their health is challenged.

To integrate the dimension of spirituality into the treatment of pain requires a partnership of healing between patient and physician, even more so than decision-making about procedural interventions, physical therapy, and mind-body techniques. If you are facing a surgical procedure without the spiritual support you need, ask friends, family, a chaplain, or a local church leader for help. Let your medical team know what you are doing and why, so they can cooperate as much as possible. Ask your physician about his or her comfort level with integrating spiritual resources in your treatment.

PRACTICING RENEWAL

When I set apart quiet time in the morning because I'm anxious about the potential land mines of the upcoming day, I practice Christian meditation to calm my spirit. Richard Foster, the Quaker author, has been my mentor.[45] One exercise he teaches involves sitting and in a rhythmical pattern breathing in the grace of God, breathing out fear, breathing in the Holy Spirit, breathing out anxiety. This practice is especially helpful with patients anticipating surgery.

The power of spiritual renewal, combined with appropriate pain treatment, was especially evident in a patient of mine suffering with complex regional pain syndrome (RSD), a sympathetic nervous system dysfunction causing agonizing neuropathic pain (of nerve origin). Jennifer Knott had RSD in two, possibly three, extremities. She was miserable and deactivated, with other health problems including bilateral mastectomies for breast cancer. A speech pathologist, Jennifer was running out of energy and spirit as she desperately sought a way to continue functioning effectively.

We tried numerous meditations, blocks, and methodologies to deal with Jennifer's neuropathic pain. She started warm water exercises, which began to make a difference. She progressed rapidly, acquired a swim coach, and started training for the Special Olympics.

Jennifer's hope for a future began to distance her from a life dominated by chronic pain and helped her revive a dormant spiritual seed. She had been raised traditional Catholic, and although she hadn't fallen away from the church it was hard for her to integrate her Catholicism effectively in managing pain. We helped her locate a Jungian psychologist, who was also a priest, to help her integrate her struggles with her spiritual growth. This, along with her swimming, enabled her to build a stronger sense of self, reasons for hope, and ways to celebrate her unique personhood.

Jennifer improved so significantly that she won several gold medals at the national Special Olympics and became a local hero in the Albuquerque newspapers. In the process of reactivation, she found a special place where she was acknowledged and applauded. She built a track record of accomplishment while continuing to deal with painful RSD. Physiologically, she progressed significantly, although intermittently she continued to need a wheelchair. She has helped other chronic pain patients reactivate themselves by finding and nurturing their spiritual center.

THE TRANSFORMING POWER OF PRAYER

Although there are many components to the spiritual life, I believe prayer is foundational. It is the movement of your spirit, and it will move you beyond somatic (body-focused) preoccupation toward the larger life that is not dominated and defined by your illness or injury. It nurtures the spirit as it quiets mind and body, strengthening the inner life just as weight-lifting builds muscle. Prayer takes as many different forms and expressions as there are individuals and beliefs, but it has proven to be consistently effective in healing and maintaining health. No one can substantiate supernatural answers to prayer, but scientists have proven that it has top-down calming effects physiologically (see chapter four). However, you don't have to understand why prayer works in order to embrace it and practice it.

Prayer is perhaps the shortest route from our society's obsession with youth, superficial beauty, and perfect health to a grounded awareness of what is truly life-giving. In his book *Living Your Dying*, Joseph Sharp comments, "When we begin to look at our spiritual practices we begin to see that their purpose is not to inoculate us from pain but to provide us with the tools with which to process and transform seemingly meaningless pain into meaningful growth."[46] Prayer is a vital way of processing pain into growth and becoming spiritually prepared to face aging, suffering, and even death.

Our impulse is to beg God to take away the pain, because that seems the only solution to the problem. We cannot see any benefit from the pain, and all we want is an end to it. When we don't have enough insight to know how or what to pray, "Thy will be done" is perhaps the best plea. As we learn the mechanisms to modulate pain and understand how it controls our moods, prayer will begin to shift us from desperate pleading into reverence for God and thankfulness for moments of less pain. What we ask for in relief of discomfort may frequently change as we grow spiritually.

For those whose pain traps them excruciatingly inside their bodies in a hellish present that seems to have neither end nor exit, prayer can open the way to an interlude of timelessness—a merciful transcendence of suffering. This experience has been described by mystics across the world's great religious traditions—Christian, Jewish, Muslim, and Hindu. It is sometimes referred to as the "eternal now" —a state of being in which the boundaries of past, present, and future melt away in the perceived union of the soul with ultimate reality or infinite being. In their analysis of the relationship between the brain and religious experience,

Eugene d'Aquili and Andrew Newberg refer to this altered state of consciousness as "absolute unitary being."[47]

Living prayerfully can help you integrate spirit, mind, and body in moving toward wholeness through the healing process. The spiritual disciplines of the ancient Christian tradition, such as fasting, meditation, silence and solitude, appointed hours for daily and nightly rites, and simple ritual petitions were developed to help weave prayer into the warp and weft of thought and action. Here is an example of praying the simple "Jesus prayer," an Eastern Orthodox practice. This quote is from Gregory of Sinai, a fourteenth-century monastic:

> Sit down alone and in silence. Lower your head, shut your eyes, breathe out gently and imagine yourself looking into your own heart. Carry your mind, that is, your thoughts, from your head to your heart. As you breathe out, say, 'Lord Jesus Christ, have mercy on me.' Say it moving your lips gently, or simply say it in your mind. Try to put all other thoughts aside. Be calm, be patient and repeat the process very frequently.

Orthodox Christians who practice this prayer regularly attest to its transforming power to move the human spirit into communion with the Divine.

One of the most vivid examples of transformation I have been privileged to witness is manifested in the life of one of my patients, an ENT surgeon about my age, whom I have known for many years. Well over ten years ago, when I first met him, he was an aggressive professional with a strong and dominant ego, very much part of mainstream society. In our early years of working together I didn't know much about him except that he was a very good surgeon. Then he went through a very difficult divorce and somewhere in the process became a Buddhist. He pursued it quite seriously, often going away on retreat for as much as a month at a time to sit with different teachers.

Quietly and gradually, this man's personality has changed. At least from all outward appearances, he is now a peaceful, gentle, reflective soul. He no longer performs as many surgeries as he used to, and he regularly takes time out to be away from the office. Those of us who have known him before and after his major life change have witnessed a metamorphosis. His practice is small, his needs are simple, and his quiet contentment is clear. In the midst of great heartache, he has found a spiritual path that is true for him, and is far more valuable than his medical practice.

Many years ago, when he was just beginning his Buddhist practice, he and I had several conversations about his intense back pain. At that time I never saw him as a patient. He had learned to manage the pain without having to undergo surgery. Several years later, however, he developed significant neck pain that radiated into his upper extremities, causing weakness and numbness in his hands and fingers that threatened his surgical career. He came to me for a cervical epidural block, which entailed placing a needle in the epidural space just behind his spinal cord and injecting medication to decrease the swelling around the cervical nerve roots. The procedure was successful in reducing the swelling, giving the nerve roots some room, and consequently easing his pain. He was able to regain strength in his hands and continue surgery, but at a more gentle pace.

He seemed remarkably calm about the whole process, and he had cancelled surgery for several months. He was viewing this event from a deeper, spiritual perspective, rather than as simply an unwanted intrusion upon his productivity. After quiet reflection, he decided to come to our pain center. He was not exceedingly hopeful that the procedure—which entailed some serious risk—would completely eliminate the pain, and he was not anxious about jumping back onto the performance treadmill of medical life. Instead, he was willing to flow with whatever was going to happen, whether it would lead him into a reduced workload or even into early retirement. In meditation, he had learned to turn over the outcome by accepting whatever spiritual path this experience would take him on. The uncertainty of being on a path he could not control was even somewhat exhilarating for him.

What struck me most about this experience was not so much that he got better because of the procedure, but the content of our conversations immediately before and after. This man had been "sitting" for ten years in daily Zen Buddhist meditation, strengthening and deepening his beliefs. When he came to me he was, like most patients, both fearful and hopeful. He feared the pain and hoped that I would be able to alleviate it. He spoke a lot about the gulf between fear and hope, two sides of the same coin. Our society, is very wrapped up in these extremes, and tends to rush from one to the other. He practiced being comfortable with staying in the space between them. He cited the Buddhist concept of the *dharmas*, pairs of opposites. Pleasure/pain is one of the dharmas, and we discussed the necessity of living with both simultaneously. Another dharma is gain/loss, which was crucial in his situation because of his surgical profession. Rather than trying to eradicate the negative extreme, he chose to occupy the middle ground, refusing to cling to one extreme over the other.

Most surgeons have strong egos. This character quality is usually considered a gift of sorts, because it requires a certain inner strength to cut into people. My friend had found a new strength in the pursuit of "egolessness," a concept common to Buddhists and Christian mystics, which involves setting aside intense personal desires so that they no longer drive thought and behavior. Two other concepts he clung to, again key to both Buddhist and Christian thought, are the impermanence of everything and the recognition of the inevitability of suffering—and its value as a source of wisdom. If the procedure was not successful and he was forced onto a different professional track, then he would accept this change as part of the impermanence of all things, and he would learn from it.

He spoke to me in a quiet, unhurried manner about how he had handled the pain during his sitting times—"leaning into" the discomfort, trying to listen closely to it. He put aside the temptation to worry anxiously about his future as a surgeon and what would happen to his income. Instead, he focused on what message the pain might have for him in the long run, rather than rushing to jump back into the professional marketplace at the earliest opportunity. My friend and colleague had discovered that the way to inner peace leads not around our fears, but through them.

WHEN SPIRITUAL PRACTICE SEEMS FUTILE

The transforming power of prayer is at work even when peace seems elusive and unattainable. Times of seeming desertion, absence, and abandonment from God appear to be universal, especially for chronic pain sufferers. Theological niceties are of little help when one is entrenched in chronic pain while at the same time in a spiritual wasteland. Sixteenth-century mystic John of the Cross called it "the dark night of the soul"; an anonymous English author identified it as "the cloud of unknowing."

Saint John of the Cross described this wilderness experience as a profound reorientation of the self, inwardly and outwardly:

> In the process of the forsaken prayer our feeling of God is hidden; there are two purifications which occur. The first strips us of dependence on exterior things. The second purification involved stripping us of dependence of the interior intelligence, pride, and charm. Our trust in all exterior and interior results is being shattered so that we learn faith in God alone. Through our barrenness of soul God is producing detachment, humility, patience, perseverance.

The Jewish and Christian scriptures are filled with stories of those who endured intense feelings of being forsaken by God: Abraham and Sarah waiting into old age for their promised offspring...Moses exiled from Egypt's splendor, waiting year after year in silence for God to show up and deliver the Israelites from slavery...the prophet Elijah, exhausted and hungry and marked for death, keeping a lonely vigil in a desolate cave...Jeremiah, lowered down into a dungeon well until he sank into the mire...Mary's vigil at her son's cross...Christ dying in agony, crying out, "My God, My God, why hast Thou forsaken me?" To feel godforsaken is a universal human experience. Pain makes us feel that this abandonment is the final truth about our lives. If we turn to God in prayer instead of turning away in despair, we will be able to see this desolation as a stage in the process of spiritual purification. The dross is being stripped away and the gold of our soul refined. However painful, it is also hopeful: we are moving toward a larger and better life. I am encouraged by this courageous prayer from the AIDS quilt: "Lead us, O God, to see a way where there is no path. Give us to hear music when our own song ceases. And when the warm touch of life forsakes us and our courage melts away, may we stumble in the darkness into Thee."[48]

In an address to the American Pain Society National meeting in 1996, Rabbi Harold S. Kushner said that in the beginning of a chronic pain experience, "our will is in struggle with God's will. We beg, we pout, we demand. We expect God to perform like a magician" to rid us of suffering.[49] After an arduous journey of pain and struggle, some people are finally able to give up begging and pleading in the relief of relinquishment. Paradoxically, this leads to freedom. The prison of pain becomes a school of surrender. Freed from desperate pleading for ourselves, we have capacity to care for others, to put their needs first, to give genuinely and joyfully. Little by little we are changed by what A. W. Tozer called a daily "crucifixion of the will."[50]

Sometimes we don't have the energy for prayer, or we're too discouraged to pray, or the circumstances aren't right and we're not ready, or we're in too much pain. But these are the times when we are most in need of prayer. Philosopher Diogenes Allen recounts the advice of Sister Basilea Schlink, the founder of a Protestant monastic order for women in the former West Germany: "When you are suffering say, 'Yes, Father,' and strength will flow into your heart.'" She offered this counsel "not as a theory, but as a description of what actually happens when we so yield."[51] It makes no difference how we feel about ourselves; when we draw near to God, even in wordless exhaustion, we open the way to experiencing how close God is to us.

Genuine healing is not always a physical change. In the divine mystery, sometimes it is a new thirst for spiritual things, a change of heart, or a peace that passes all understanding. Some miracles are visible only to the eyes of the spirit. Developing this inner vision is a form of renewing the spirit.

PRAYER BEHAVIOR VERSUS PAIN BEHAVIOR

One noticeable effect of spiritual renewal is the movement from pain behavior to prayer behavior. Margaret Mead accurately observed that our society has moved from being task-based to entertainment-based. This shift breeds passivity in many areas of life, and it shows up clearly in patients who are not used to being asked to contribute to their healing. Most of Western society looks to medicines, operations, and procedures for healing. Involvement in exercise, diet change, prayer, and methodical cognitive skills is seldom invoked as primary in the healing process.

Prayer behavior is virtually the opposite of pain behavior. In pain medicine, we refer to pain behavior as action that seeks help and sympathy. Limping, grimacing, and whining are manifestations of distress that exaggerate the pain.

We all have pain behavior. Mine often follows when I have been up all night in surgery. I can make my eyes look deeper within their sockets so I *really* look exhausted. I go around the hospital projecting an image of self-sacrifice, but inwardly seeking sympathy for my hard work and fatigue. We all do this to some degree, but chronic pain patients create an aura of pain behavior around their persona. If this can be pointed out in a humorous way, patients are less likely to assume the dependent posture that distances them from healthcare providers and their relatives. Occasionally we take videos of patients exhibiting pain behavior and play the tapes for them. They are often shocked, but the exercise helps them make adjustments to move beyond the pain.

Prayer focuses upward and outward, away from the body. Pain behavior focuses inward on the body. Prayer moves toward others, interceding on their behalf. It is often selfless rather than self-centered. Prayer is a way of turning over of control. Pain behavior is a way of seeking control. Prayer behavior is characterized by mature expressions of love and service. Pain behavior demands love and service from others. Prayer behavior seeks truth, clarity, and honesty. Pain behavior is mired in deception, dissolution, and disappointment.

One of my beloved patients is Sister Mary Joaquin, a nun at a monastery in a very beautiful part of New Mexico on the Chama River, thirteen miles from paved roads. She suffers from a connective tissue disease, a very rare type of rheumatoid arthritis called CREST syndrome. She has many problems associated with it, including complications that have affected her heart rate, crippled her hands and her back, and left her in a great deal of pain. She has been through much adversity in her life, and she continues to teach me.

Sister often enters her prayer chamber by walking across a meadow to the primitive chapel of Christ in the Desert to meditate on the crucified Christ. If she has pain in her hip or back, she looks at the hip or back of the body on the huge crucifix and turns the pain over to Jesus. If her hands are especially painful, she gazes on the nailed hands of Jesus on the cross, meditating on the suffering he experienced. It seems to her as if Jesus is able to take some of the pain from her.

Sister practices a Catholic tradition of suffering for others: a spiritual acceptance of others' burdens while giving to them health. Sister once witnessed the miracle of an elderly woman giving her sight to an almost blind young person. She practices taking in other people's suffering, breathing in the pain and breathing out healing, much like the Buddhist practice of tonglen.

Because of her personal adversity, Sister can suffer more easily for others in prayer and meditation. She has known many people in chronic pain who are unable to get outside themselves, making it very difficult for others to take care of them. She has learned how to focus on Jesus in meditation in order to keep from being enveloped when the pain of the far-advanced CREST syndrome disease threatens to overwhelm her. This practice frees her from becoming lost in her own suffering, so that she can focus on others in need.

Sister recalled the story of Mother Teresa changing a dressing on a leper, while an interviewing journalist exclaimed that he wouldn't take that dressing off for a million dollars. Mother Teresa turned to him and said she wouldn't do it for a million dollars either—only for Jesus. Sister admired the way Mother Teresa's life was filled with Jesus. She did not want the world's attention—she seemed to have attained egolessness.

Sister Joaquin sees many parallels among the major religious traditions and believes there are universal truths present in all of them. The purifying effect of pain is one of them: "When I have less pain," she told me, "my meditation is less effective. The greater my pain, the more effective I am in meditation." She no longer asks for relief of her pain, because she views it as a gift enabling her to focus on others' suffering in prayer and meditation.

Sister endured a period of significant depression when she could not find a way in her elderly years to be productive. The only way she was able to get through it was by meditating on the sufferings of Christ. Eventually, her depression began to lift as she was able to turn her pain over to Jesus and allow it to become a vehicle through which healing love could flow to others. The life of the spirit does not yield steady upward progress, she feels. All of us have times when we feel far from God, and when prayer and meditation seem useless. In fact, the longer we live, the more these times of distance will characterize our experience. Interludes of feeling God's presence in a close and intimate way are precious and few.

Recently, Sister returned to the pain center with worsened arthritis. She had pain in her lower back and radiating down one leg. Under flouoroscopy (a dynamic x-ray process), her spine appeared profoundly arthritic. My job was to try to locate a specific nerve, block it, and put some medication around that area to decrease the nerve inflammation. It was an arduous process, and Sister, in her seventy-eight years, was peaceful and calm during the hour-long procedure. It was difficult for me to place needles accurately, even with the latest fluoroscopic technology. I was doubtful that this would be a long-term solution for her pain, but the surgeons were wary of performing any more operations on her because of her age and medical problems.

We were able to relieve the pain almost entirely for five days, and then it came lunging back. You might expect that temporary relief would be followed by despair in such a case; Sister viewed the five days as a wonderful gift. She wrote to me that she was able once again to be almost pain-free, and to take a much-needed breather from the severity of the physical suffering and the intensity of her meditative prayer. It was as if the field were able to lie fallow for a brief period of time, giving her strength to re-enter the strenuous process of enduring the pain and struggling in prayer for those who suffer. My colleagues and I are debating whether to do the procedure again, but I am struck by how she values both the pain and the respite from it.

RECOVERING WHOLENESS

In childhood we often experience a sense of wholeness that we later lose in adulthood. A child has not yet learned to ignore some parts of reality in order to pursue others; there is an unselfconscious unity. I find that when I ask people to allow their child to revisit their adult, it puts them in touch with the vulnerable and tender parts of themselves they have starved out or left behind. Recovering these lost parts is what helps them move toward a larger sense of what life is about, to reconnect with what is most important.

There may be some deep spiritual truth from childhood that has lain dormant for years. Perhaps letting the child revisit the adult will reawaken some authentic truths for you. Seeking ways to grow spiritually will strengthen you for growing through pain instead of being diminished and defeated by it. You may not recover the physical wholeness you had before the pain set in, but as you strengthen your spirit you will most likely recover a sense of what you thought had been lost to you forever.

In the healing process, most patients have a strong sense of "returning" to what they once believed but lost faith in, to a sense of self that had been neglected or buried by the pressures of life and the crisis of declining health, to a simple happiness and peace they have not experienced since the best moments of their childhood.

One of my patients was a very attractive woman in her late thirties with intellectual prowess to match her physical beauty. After graduating from Harvard Business School she went on to earn a doctorate in nuclear physics. Her regular work-outs in the gym had sculpted her body to a physique that could grace magazine covers. She had all the gifts that our society prizes and she worked very hard to make sure she excelled in all of them. Her husband was an accomplished professional as well, and although their busy lives did not afford much time for nurturing the marriage, they had managed to add two children. Even their family unit seemed a mark of their achievement.

Her constant success-seeking began foundering, however, with severe migraine headaches. They had been her Achilles' heel all her adult life, but now they were steadily worsening, eroding her productivity. She'd been to clinics all over the country, especially in California, and tried virtually every new treatment known or proposed.

I faced my initial appointment with her with some trepidation, wondering if I would be expected to figure out some new pharmacological intervention that all of California had not been able to come up with. She was very intent upon finding a medication that would keep her on the path of productivity. Our initial discussions revealed that she had done virtually nothing in the area of mind-body work, because she did not believe it would be much help. She was extremely concrete in her thinking, and mind-body techniques did not seem very concrete to her.

She agreed to give this direction a try, however, when I explained to her how processes such as hypnosis, biofeedback, and relaxation exercises directly affect the interrelation of the brain and the nervous system in turning the volume of pain up or down. I also referred her to a behavioral psychologist from England, practicing in Albuquerque, who was especially gifted at working in concrete ways.

In a very short period of time she began to notice a positive difference. I was especially intrigued by her description of "feeling" her mental pathways. An inveterate perfectionist, she was given to fits of road rage with other drivers. After a few sessions of mind-body work, she became sensitized to what was happening in her thought patterns during these episodes. She began to notice other contexts in which these same brain pathways went on red alert: impatience with others when they did not perform, frustration with herself when she failed to attain her high standards. Her work on cognitive thought patterns gave her a new understanding of the mechanistic ways she was triggering or reinforcing her headaches. For the first time in her life, she began to feel hopeful about the possibility that she could do something to help reverse these headaches.

She had very few women friends; her image of perfection had kept others at a distance from her. She began to experience endearment directed toward her not-so-perfect self. There began to be a noticeable body-mind shift. After she acknowledged the body-mind connection, we began to explore the possibilities of the body-spirit connection, to consider moving from her left-brain physicist, business school mentality to her right-brain vulnerability and her childhood desire to be in touch with spiritual things.

I told her that just as it requires hard work at the health spa to change the way you look, it it takes a lot of regular work to experience psychological and spiritual growth. She recognizes that if she is going to change that physiological response of headaches, she is going to have to be comfortable with the mystery that psychology and spirituality can definitely affect physical things. She has an enormous amount of energy—as she redirects some of it in acknowledging that spirituality is as important as concrete physical realities, she will make a big difference in her headaches.

She is being vulnerable in admitting that the spiritual realm is new to her—not only that, but she recognizes that she has missed so much in this area by focusing so exclusively on her professional accomplishments and her physical beauty. She has begun to realize that reconnecting with her spirituality can help her with the body-mind connection. She can actually visualize the shifting of the intensity of her headaches and her responses to life. Her needs for affection, for people to like her for who she is rather than for what she does, are now being met. She practices showing vulnerability and has been rewarded with warmer reactions from people than she has ever received before—strokes she has really needed.

However you select your spiritual path, learn to acknowledge and reinforce it throughout the day. The ordinary, everyday moments of life offer us numerous opportunities to work on our spirits—waiting at the red light, in the doctor's office, in line at the grocery store. This is the ground God meets you on: where your pain meets you.

STEPS FOR THE PATH:
ENERGIZING THE POWER OF THE SPIRIT

1. *Today, I would rate my general pain level as:*

   0   1   2   3   4   5   6   7   8   9   10
   pain free   excruciating pain

2. *Do you have any experience with practicing a daily spiritual discipline such as prayer, quiet reflection, or meditative reading? How has it helped you deal with your pain?*

3. *Scientific advances in Western medicine have increased exponentially the options for treatment. But these advances have also tended to exclude any appreciation for the mystery of healing. Consider the difference between "cure" and "healing."*

4. *One way to re-energize the spirit is to change how you think of yourself. You are no longer an injured person, but a well person with a problem. Take an inventory of your mental, physical, and spiritual health. You will find that what is right with your body is far greater than what is wrong with it.*

5. *In what ways can you practice your own authentic spirituality in the "little whiles" of life—waiting in the doctor's office, stalled in traffic, starting or ending your day, embarking on a difficult task?*

CHAPTER SEVEN

EMBRACING THE PARADOX OF PAIN

With the help of the thorn in my foot,
I spring higher than anyone with sound feet.

—SØREN KIERKEGAARD

A NOTHER PATIENT IS DYING in the hospital. Sue is an attractive forty-eight-year-old Santa Fe resident, well to do, with three healthy adult children. She and her ex-husband, both successful in business, divorced ten years earlier. Sue did well following the end of the marriage, found a male companion, and seemed to be enjoying the good life. Then she was diagnosed with advanced cancer of the colon.

Sue was bounced all around New Mexico and Texas in efforts to fight this difficult cancer. The medical approaches were definitely conventional Western: surgery, chemotherapy, and radiation. As she ran out of options, her children flew home to help care for her, administering her daily medication and trying to make her comfortable while the disease progressed. Her male friend disappeared, and her children remained by her side giving her round-the-clock care.

Sue's condition rapidly worsened, and she had to be readmitted to the hospital. A psychologist who had seen the children during their parents' divorce called me and asked me to visit with the four of them for counsel on pain relief.

No one wanted Sue to die in the hospital, but she was heavily medicated and often incoherent. The children were telescoping a lifetime of emotions into this single event, cramming for finals without having taken the course. They had virtually no support system—their father was long gone, at least emotionally, and the boyfriend had disappeared. Their attractive mother, among the elite few with all the looks, power, and material things anyone could want, was dying, and all the medical knowledge money could buy could not help her. It was a dizzyingly steep fall from grace.

By the time I saw her after her hospital admission, some of the medication seemed to be clearing from her system, and she was noticeably brighter-eyed. I took her children into the hall and told them their counselor had called me. We discussed the importance of hospice, which they'd already begun to explore, and the option of bringing their mother home. But how do affluent young adults with a mother who is dying deal with that responsibility, having had no preparation for it? In our society, we are typically shielded from the graphic reality of death, even with family-friendly facilities. Nothing about the lives of these young people, who were so familiar with the things others envy, had helped them face such a moment as this. Fortunately they were very kind-hearted and open; it was clear they were learning at a breakneck pace.

I spoke with Sue's children about non-denominational spirituality and how important it was for them to continue therapy for closure. To honor their mother and grow from this experience, they needed to see it as an opportunity to develop inner resources they didn't know they had, to explore spaces in their mind where they hadn't been before, to become more profound people with a deeper empathy for others. It was an opportunity for them to reach within, to find a philosophical or spiritual beginning. With tears in their eyes, they listened intently about these new concepts. My psychologist friend continued to work with them on the loss of a parent, on how to harvest this very difficult experience for their own growth.

Nobody would choose the pain of watching a parent die, but it is a sure catapult out of a pleasure-seeking orientation to a far more profound and enduring approach to life. In this respect, those who have not been close to pain and suffering are at a disadvantage, because in a spiritual sense their lives are constricted.

Sue's children had an opportunity to honor their mother by helping her pass beyond this life. She was able to see in their faces a maturing gentleness and peace, which gave her a sense of completion of her task as a mother. They, in turn, were more able to celebrate her life as well as her death when the time came.

To move beyond merely coping with pain to integrating the pain experience within a larger life, it is necessary to come to grips with a fundamental paradox: *the very thing that is supposed to help you may make the pain worse, and what you think will hurt you may be the thing that frees you from a pain-dominated life.* Leveraging the pain paradox for renewing hope and forging a new vision for day-to-day life requires foundational shifts in attitudes and perspectives.

REVERSING EXPECTATIONS

One of the first significant tasks in embracing this paradox is *reversing expectations*. By the time patients arrive at the pain center, they are often weighed down by a sense of therapeutic and personal failure. The system has failed them. The medical establishment doesn't know what to do with them anymore. Friends and acquaintances with the luxury of easy health have grown impatient and frustrated, wondering why they can't just get past the problem and move on with their lives. Intensifying their discouragement is the recognition that the very steps taken to solve the problem seem only to have made it worse.

The physiology of pain has made us aware of the rebound trap—a physical reaction to an intervention (usually repeated excessively) that has exactly the opposite effect of what the treatment is intended to produce. The rebound phenomenon was first described and most clearly developed in regard to recurring headaches. Taking a narcotic for recurrent headaches may alleviate the pain momentarily, but it will saturate receptor sites in the brain and therefore ensure the reappearance of the headache. If the receptor sites can be desaturated, the headaches can be down-regulated. Paradoxically, too much of a good thing can turn into a bad thing when the body conditions itself around the intervention.

For pain patients, recovery often starts with the recognition that they will have to let go of their expectations for what they thought would help them. At first this appears to be a very discouraging threshold to cross. But it is most often the entry point to discovering how to find genuine help. It represents an opportunity for pain sufferers to make a choice. Either they can go back to old ways of coping with the pain, which even if ineffective are at least comfortingly familiar, or they can brave the unfamiliar and move ahead into new ways of looking at their future. Virtually every day we lead people to this decision point. Some turn back in fear. Others summon the courage to move forward within hope. These individuals are learning to embrace the pain paradox.

Our culture is so fixated on eliminating discomfort and obtaining immediate gratification that the pain paradox is a new concept for many. We think that our technical expertise will continue to offer endless improvements to our quality of life. We presume that we can take control of our destiny, take charge of our health, and postpone our aging. We deserve a pain-free existence, and we follow whatever or whoever promises to bring us closer to achieving it. If we have an ache, we take a pill to make it go away. If the ache persists, we take more pills.

Productive, task-oriented people often measure their personal worth according to their accomplishments. When chronic pain strikes, they are at high risk for depression, because once they fall off the roller coaster of achievement, their self-esteem comes tumbling down. Ironically, those with power in our society are often the most fragile when they confront loss of control from pain. Receiving a disability check, for example, is both a blessing and a curse. It affords financial relief, but it can be psychologically limiting in reversing the concept of personal worth built around vocational productivity and accomplishment.

My Navajo friend Norman Yazzie observes that even education can be a liability, because it can lead to trusting the written word more than what is written in the heart. Education can pull a person's life off-center into spiritual imbalance when it confuses wisdom with acquiring information or with achieving successive levels of academic accomplishment. Native Americans often laugh at our conventional thirst for status and power, because it is so opposed to a life of harmony. De-humanization and de-spiritualization go hand in hand with a culture that honors power, money, and technology. In recent years it has become trendy to seek an integrated or holistic approach to life, but Native American culture has always had the concept of harmony and balance embedded in its mores. Suffering is not an unexpected intrusion on the good life, but simply one more step toward completing the cycle of earthly life and moving on to the spirit world.

Our cultural expectations influence our response to the anger and loss that accompany pain. Depression is often the result—the suppression of anger toward the apparent unfairness of life's circumstances, at family members who have trouble understanding the pain experience, and at God for allowing bad things to happen. Pain sufferers are also vulnerable to experiencing loss of physical capacity, loss in their ability to maintain friendships, and loss of self-confidence. These losses can be overwhelming, which may lead to depression as well.

Our pain-phobic society can learn from the Native Americans who lived here in Santa Fe five hundred years before the Spaniards came. We avoid pain at any price; Native Americans quietly embrace it as a teacher. Which is the more advanced society—the one that shoves pain under the rug, and pays a severe price for doing so? And which is the so-called primitive society—the one that welcomes suffering as a friend, enhancing the journey through life?

Our assumption that technological prowess can protect us from pain and illness is built on the illusion that we are in control. Again and again we learn the hard lesson that we are not. Non-smokers contract lung cancer. People who eat nutritionally, exercise regularly, and nurture their inner life find their biopsies coming back positive for terminal cancer.

In this world, no one is immune to pain and suffering, not even the spiritually-enlightened heroes of our religious traditions. The Old Testament figure Job, an innocent man, never did receive an explanation from God for why he had been subjected to unfathomable suffering. Jesus Christ was executed on a cross. Buddha, the Awakened One, died from food poisoning. Catholic mystic Terésa of Ávila was afflicted with crippling arthritis. Ultimately, the presence of pain is a mystery. In this life we see through a glass darkly, said the apostle Paul, but one day we will see clearly.[52]

For most of us, the great trials of life will simply leave us with a lot of unanswered questions. As we begin to let go of the demand for answers, the anxious thoughts of the mind may yield to the strengthening of the spirit.

UNDERSTANDING THE PLEASURE-PAIN RELATIONSHIP

Another shift that most people in our culture are required to make in order to leverage the pain paradox is overcoming the artificial separation of pleasure and pain. We blithely assume that pleasure is good and pain is bad, so we pursue the one and flee from the other. But pain is not punishment, and pleasure is not reward, despite our persistent attempts to treat them as such. Where in Western society did we ever get the idea that we can have pleasure without pain? Birth is painful as well as delightful. The painful reality of death may bring with it a pleasurable release, an exhilarating closure. Pleasure and pain are inextricably linked.

Eugene d'Aquili and Andrew Newberg have identified what they call "cognitive operators" to describe specific functions performed by specific parts of the brain. These operators allow the mind to think, feel, experience, order, and interpret the world. One of them is the binary operator, which derives meaning by establishing "dyads," or pairs of opposites: good and evil, right and wrong, and justice and injustice. The description of these dyads provides an ideal depiction of the pleasure/pain relationship:

> It is important to note that each opposite in the dyad, in some ways, derives its meaning from its contrast with the other opposite. In this sense, the opposites do not stand completely on their own, but require each other in order to define themselves individually.[53]

Patients instantly understand "the pleasure/pain syndrome" when I describe the simple example of scratching an itch: it feels good while it hurts even more. The same is true with deep massage. Marathon runners push their bodies through pain and experience pleasure simultaneously, from the release of endorphins and the ecstasy of accomplishment. Leonardo da Vinci understood this paradox five hundred years ago when he drew the "Allegory of Pleasure and Pain," depicting twins joined at the waist.

Historians of the Christian church have observed that the growth and vitality of the church tends to be in inverse proportion to the comfort level of its social context. When the emperor Constantine legitimized Christian faith in the fourth century, the energy of the persecuted church subsided into the complacency of the publicly accepted church. Oppression and hardship seem to accelerate rather than diminish the fervor of commitment.

I often wonder what benefits we have given up in our cultural preoccupation with comfort and luxury. Growing up, I listened to my relatives swapping stories about life during the Great Depression and World Wars I and II. They also discussed the hardships of enduring frigid high-mountain winters without central heating. My mother and her siblings drove a buckboard many miles to school in the coldest part of Colorado, with bricks heated in the wood-burning stove placed at their feet. But my parents, aunts, and uncles talked about these experiences as fond memories, as if the difficulties had inspired rather than defeated them.

My generational stories include the war in Vietnam. One of the most difficult experiences I endured was serving as commanding officer of a mobile medical clearing station in the central highlands of Vietnam. We operated under constant threat of being overrun at any moment by the Vietcong. Our medical unit tended to any and all wounded—American and South Vietnamese soldiers, Vietcong and North Vietnamese soldiers, civilians, and Montagnards. Fear co-existed with excitement in the midst of this severe situation. Abandoning myself to the work despite the imminent dangers, I was surprised by feelings of intense joy. Although there was much about that time in my life I am glad to have behind me, there is much I miss about it as well.

Today in the United States, when unprecedented numbers of people are living the so-called American dream, the good life does not always seem quite as good as promised. Why the deep irony that affluence in our Western society seems to make pleasure more difficult to reach? Certainly, no society has succeeded so well in trying to eliminate pain and to exploit pleasure. Yet happiness still seems elusive. Perhaps the more a society tries to eliminate pain, the less it is able to cope with the suffering that remains.

In our technologically advanced society we consider discomfort a problem to be solved, while cultures more attuned to natural rhythms tend to have a more balanced view of life's mix of pleasure and pain. This leaves us less prepared to face adversity when it strikes. Thanks to a gifted and determined teacher, Helen Keller broke through the imprisonment of her severe disabilities to provide wisdom and inspiration that no disability-free person could attain. "I am grateful for my handicap," she declared, "for through it I found my world, my self, and my God." She was insightful enough to recognize the dangers of complacency in a world lulled by comfort: "As the eagle was killed by the arrow winged with his own feather," she observed, "so the hand of the world is wounded by its own skill."

I have come to appreciate the Buddhist concept of *tonglen* as one of the best ways to avoid the swings between pain-phobia and pleasure-seeking extremes. Tonglen is a practice of taking in pain and sending out pleasure. For example, in the presence of a pain sufferer, it might mean quietly "breathing in" that person's pain and "breathing out" healing. Connecting in this way with the suffering around us helps to liberate us from self-centered patterns and awaken to compassion.

How little we realize what suffering we inflict upon ourselves by investing so heavily in protecting our own interests. When somebody criticizes us and we feel insulted, we mobilize our resources to defend against the attack. This doesn't do much except focus our attention all the more on the perceived insult, giving it greater power over us. When pain strikes, we focus all our energies on eliminating it, which paradoxically often intensifies it. If we enlarged our frame of reference to include the pain of others, allowing our pain to sensitize us to others' suffering, this movement away from self-absorption can actually lessen our pain—and that of others, as we offer an understanding and caring presence to them.

Buddhists emphasize seeking the middle ground as an antidote to being dominated by extremes. Instead of swinging wildly between pain and pleasure, and fear and hope, the Buddhist accepts the paradoxical existence of these opposites. Since suffering is an inevitable but impermanent reality, it is important to be gentle with oneself and others, to avoid insisting that life unfold according to one's personal agenda, and to refuse to act on the clamorous demands of the ego. In this way, energies can be redirected from the futile attempt to eradicate pain to finding harmony in the coexistence of pain and pleasure.

My friend Guru Terath Kaur Khalsa, a Sikh psychologist, believes that our body cells store memories of our experiences, including those of past lives. For the Sikhs, each person is a trinity of body, mind, and spirit. Since what is stored in the body affects the mind and spirit, these memories can help or hinder the way we respond to pain. Guru Khalsa advises that we get to know our pain and that we befriend it as a path to understanding the lessons we need to learn in order to go home to God. If we suppress our pain or try to avoid it, the consequences will include remaining in the cycles of this earthly realm until the soul is ready to move on.

The Sikhs' approach to pain has parallels in their views of death. Much like some Native Americans, Sikhs believe you should not wait until your death to practice dying. In their tradition, after deeply meditating then lying back to relax, there is a sense of the body dropping and the soul traveling. This meditation may serve as practice for death—a way to face it and greet it instead of avoiding it in fear.

Both Western and Eastern spiritual traditions are steeped in wisdom principles arising from suffering. Zen Buddhists "lean into" their pain. Christians revere Christ on the cross—and, in addition to claiming his sacrifice as atonement for their sins, they draw comfort from the companionship of God in suffering. In both religions, suffering itself is impermanent, and perfect peace awaits us beyond this earthly life. Therefore, the acceptance of suffering now is not a capitulation to despair, but a quiet recognition that pain does not have power to define life—rather, life defines pain by placing it within a larger framework. It is possible to find serenity between the extremes of fear and hope. It is possible for suffering to be endured not as the end of hope, but as a path toward healing.

LISTENING TO INNER KNOWING

Cultural conditioning is especially difficult to overcome in an outer-directed society that values conformity over integrity. In our consumer mindset, we have ceded enormous control of our values and decisions to the dictates of the marketplace. Market values inevitably reinforce a tendency toward the acquisition of material goods, the enhancement of personal status as defined by fluctuating social values, and the increase of power in wielding control over the instruments of commerce. Those who are socially disadvantaged by the encumbrances of pain are, therefore, consistently de-valued. This chips away at their self-confidence, making it all the more difficult to trust in their own gut instincts for finding a way forward through the pain to a productive and meaningful life.

I emphasize the importance of inner knowing with my patients because I believe that, on one level or another, we all know the truth about ourselves. Accessing this knowledge can be a crucial component of the healing process. Apparently healthy people will sometimes have a premonition when they go to a doctor about a disease that will be diagnosed. Pregnant women sometimes have a sure sense of their unborn baby's gender. Elderly people have been known to predict the time and season of their death, even down to the day and location.

Our bodies are rich repositories of information about what is going on within. Sometimes the data is transmitted consciously to the mind through specific and identifiable symptoms, but other times the body buries information for years, especially in cases of extreme trauma, until mind and spirit are capable of recognizing and assimilating the information. Other times the body's wisdom is manifested in a persistent, nagging sense of something unidentifiable, like continually catching a glimpse of something in our peripheral vision that we know is there but can't quite identify.

In 1985 I went in for a routine chest x-ray to comply with an insurance exam, feeling deep anxiety. When the film came back showing that my heart was markedly enlarged, it gave a name to my restless fear. Faced with the life-threatening diagnosis of a faulty mitral valve, I pored over the literature to research treatment options while relying on my sense of inner knowing, guided by prayer, to direct my choices.

Inner knowing is extremely important for patients who must make difficult decisions or guide their healthcare providers in pursuing treatment options. This was the discovery made by Janet Nyberg, R.N., author of Chronic Pain, Finding a Life Worth Living. A nurse afflicted with failed back syndrome, Nyberg wrote about the frustrations of trying to find treatment for her chronic pain. "When the cure fails," she observed, "physicians become insecure, hesitant, and vague; they look for ways to blame the patient rather than themselves."[55] Defensive physicians are often people with a precarious sense of self-esteem who have worked very hard to be successful. Because they measure their acceptance by their accomplishment, it is personally very threatening to feel unsuccessful.

To make matters worse, Nyberg found that insurance companies treat pain patients as if they are dishonest, malingerers, or leeches on the healthcare system. This only aggravates depression and a sense of helplessness. "What this crazy system does," she concluded, "is make those who suffer (the truly ill) suffer even more by being treated like enemies for needing healthcare."[56]

After more than ten years of procedures, surgeries, dashed hopes, and depression, Nyberg's downward cycle culminated in a suicide attempt. Previously a self-proclaimed "born again" Christian, she had perhaps fallen harder than those without a strong faith because now even God had deserted her—the ultimate abandonment.

Nyberg began to emerge from the deadly control of pain only after turning her focus more directly to the care of her soul. She formed a pain support group with a ten-step program intended to move a member from a "patient" to a "person." The cornerstone of the support group was that God or a greater being cares individually for each person, and this gave her a renewed sense of hope. "As my anger with God dimin-ished...," she wrote, "I began to feel anew that God would always have a place in my heart. I felt that I needed to pay more attention to the healing of my soul. I began reading the Bible and other religious books and to pray that God would have a bigger impact on my life."[57]

Developing this new orientation was a long, intense, and difficult process. Nyberg was forced to rely on her own inner knowing because all the conventional treatments had left her high and dry. "Reconstructing a life worth living is a slow, ongoing process of 'becoming'—of finding inside oneself a new person who can learn to live a meaningful life in spite of the pain,"[58] she observed. She discovered that the two most vital but difficult steps were letting go of previous misconceptions, giving up attempts to change things that cannot be changed, and moving on—making a conscious choice to go forward with a new view.

Pain patients sometimes know better than their families and even their healthcare providers what kind of support they need—and what kind of help is not helpful. The self-help health movement has made tremen-dous strides in offsetting the imperialism of traditional medicine. We have become more aware than ever before of the need to be proactive in taking responsibility for our well-being rather than leaving it up to the professionals.

Nevertheless, those in chronic pain are by definition operating with a deficit of emotional and physical resources, which makes it harder to take initiative especially when it cuts against the grain of prevailing opinion. They are often viewed with suspicion or impatience, which can be very intimidating to the pain sufferer.

Standing firm on the basis of personal conviction when you are up against conventional "wisdom" is a difficult counter-move. But this is precisely when inner knowing may be the most valuable tool in your arsenal. Your body may be telling you that it doesn't need the operation everyone else thinks you should have. Or you may be realizing deep within yourself that instead of muscling your way through the pain or trying to get your mind off of it, you need to listen to it even more intently. The pain may be a signal of something happening within you at a deeper level. You will need to examine and understand that deeper reality in order to make choices that are consistent with it—instead of accepting the choices others may try to make for you, force-fitting a preconceived framework around your unique circumstances.

Pain will give you an opportunity to rely on inner knowing, especially in a society that avoids and dismisses it. It will telescope this knowledge for you, fine-tuning the flow of communication through body, mind, and spirit—from cellular, to mental and emotional, and to spiritual levels. Even when your inner voice has been battered by illness or trauma, it can still be your most precious and valuable teacher. For Christians, this voice may be the whisper of the Holy Spirit. For others, it may be simply "a higher power." The non-religious might think of it simply as their own spirit within, articulating meaning and purpose in the midst of difficult circumstances.

Regardless of the source you ascribe to your inner knowing, do not devalue it. Social pressures may make you feel as if you are chasing an illusion. The frenetic demands of everyday life will suggest that it is foolish to take time to listen for an inner voice—there is so much that obviously needs your attention. But the greater illusion is that the spirit, or Spirit, is not there. I believe it is a false message that keeps us entrapped. Mistaking volume for significance, we tend to be distracted by the loudest voices. Paradoxically, the most important messages often come to us in the most quiet and personal ways.

TAKING A TIME-OUT

Recognizing the paradox at the heart of pain is not easy to do when you are caught up in the grind of daily survival. Just as pain telescopes the process of inner knowing, it also calibrates the attention span. Maintaining a broad perspective across the landscape of our lives is impossible when one particular section is demanding all our attention and energy now. In this respect, the intrusion of pain forces us to take a time-out from life as usual. As Paul Brand observed, "pain shrinks time to the present moment...you feel miserable enough to stop whatever you're doing and pay attention."[59]

Pain unmakes a person's world. It disrupts the rhythms of daily life which pain-free people have the luxury of experiencing as routine, rituals that help define reality as safe and predictable. "The mind is its own place," declared the poet John Milton, "and in itself can make a heav'n of hell, a hell of heav'n."[60] Acute pain can be so disorienting that it is wise to prepare for it in advance by weaving a safety net of responses for modifying the pain and a support system to prevent isolation.

Belden Lane has written eloquently of the relationship between landscape and spirituality. He likens the intrusion of suffering to being thrust involuntarily into a desert experience:

> The desert as metaphor is that uncharted terrain beyond the edges of the seemingly secure and structured world in which we take such confidence, a world of affluence and order we cannot imagine ever ending. Yet it does. And at the point where the world begins to crack, where brokenness and disorientation suddenly overtake us, there we step into the wide, silent plains of a desert we had never known existed.[61]

The unmaking of everyday reality is a painful stripping process. But it can also become a clarifying process, enabling us to see with sharpened vision what is essential to our existence.

If you have ever hiked in the desert, you know the sensation of being in an environment pared down to a few primal elements: blindingly intense light …heat so overpowering it seems to vacuum the moisture from your body …still air broken only by occasional sounds—a lizard scraping across the sand, the rustle of a bird in the brush, or the cry of a hawk circling far overhead. No longer distracted by the clutter of routine existence, your senses take on a heightened awareness of your surroundings. You realize there are only a few things you need for survival: enough water to keep from being desiccated by the heat; sufficient food to fuel your body to keep moving; and protective clothing to shield you from the burning presence of the sun during the day and the freezing absence of it at night. Mind and body telescope all concerns down to the acute awareness of how much your life depends upon these few essentials.

The desert experience of pain is an enforced sojourn away from the familiar landscape of life-as-usual. It narrows the field of vision while it sharpens what remains in the sights. Gone are the things you thought you needed. You are thrust into an environment that has ruthlessly pared them away. There are only a few things necessary: enough relief from the pain so that you can develop the ability to cope with it; help from those who know how to guide you toward healing; and sufficient personal support to keep you traversing this alien landscape instead of dropping in your tracks from exhaustion and discouragement.

If you drive east or west across New Mexico on Interstate 40, you will see a sparse, rather foreboding landscape. Although the desert looks dry and barren, it is richly populated with many species of plants and animals. The native peoples—Pueblo, Navajo, and Apache—chose to settle here. For them, the desert was no wasteland but a richly productive source of spiritual and physical nurture.

The desert has always beckoned those seeking relief from the noise and clutter of society. In New Mexico it is a welcome environment for artists, drawn by the dramatic lighting, vibrant colors, vast spaces, and a 360 degree view of the horizon. In ancient times, Christian monastics chose the solitude of the desert to avoid the distractions of crowded towns. In the desert, they were able to focus single-mindedly on spiritual pursuits. "Society...was regarded [by the Desert Fathers] as a shipwreck from which each single individual man had to swim for his life," wrote Thomas Merton. "These were men who believed that to let oneself drift along, passively accepting the tenets and values of what they knew as society, was purely and simply a disaster."[62]

The landscape of the desert calls us to cut back on our over-stimulated routines and focus more directly on the few things of true importance. The sparseness of visual stimuli invites deeper contemplation. Unlike being in the dense lushness of a woodland forest, in the desert the eye is naturally drawn to one object at a time—the feathery green of a creosote bush, the large dried pods of a yucca plant, or the tilt of a tumbleweed blown suddenly across the path. This effect suggests a simpler and more reflective life—a peaceful way of living.

I think of the desert side of the human person as the arid, difficult, pensive dimension, in contrast to Carl Jung's dark side, which refers to the negative and destructive aspects of personality. Illness plunges us into the desert dimension, but it can open up spaces in the mind and heart that are new and stretching. Just as time away in the desert can have a purifying effect, so the forced retreat of pain can lead to a renewed perspective.

I like to ask my patients to visualize looking at something so intently they lose sight of everything else. Then I ask them to imagine taking a step back and looking at it from high above, like watching an anthill while standing up straight instead of crouching down to peer closely at it. This is what I ask them to do with the pain experience: instead of being absorbed by it, just notice it in a disengaged way. Observe without making value judgments or analyzing: simply become aware. When Pema Chödrön teaches basic sitting meditation, she advises giving up on trying to control runaway thoughts by simply labeling them as you say the word, "thinking."[63] If you let your mind run with anxiety about your pain experience, unable to separate yourself from the pain and identifying totally with it, you are likely to intensify your pain.

Standing back to look at your life is a hidden benefit of the enforced time-out, or desert sojourn, of the pain experience. It is an extended break from being immersed in, and distracted by, everyday demands. Pain is not the only circumstance that brings this about. Sometimes a major event will do this for you: a family or health circumstance will force a change in patterns of behavior that may allow you to see from a distance what you might otherwise never have recognized. To do this purposefully, as with a sabbatical, can be even more effective. A pain patient does not do this by choice, however; it arises from desperation. At the extreme end, the time-out may be permanent, in the ultimate escape of suicide. Becoming involved in service to others can help offset the desperation by putting personal experience in perspective.

Viewing pain as a time-out from life as usual can be a profound embrace of the pain paradox. Some people discover entirely new ways of orienting their lives in response to the trauma of illness and physical suffering. In Christian tradition, the term "calling" is often used to describe a God-given vocation or central purpose around which one's life is oriented. Our busy, task-oriented society affords few built-in opportunities to stand apart and reflect quietly upon what we are doing and why we are doing it. Most of us don't take time out to look at our lives unless some event has disrupted it. Chronic pain patients have an opportunity to focus on what they believe is essential—and, in the process, perhaps to find a new sense of "calling." Being forced to stop and examine our lives closely may be a blessing, much like discovering new strength in a time of testing that reveals we are able to do or sustain more than we thought ourselves capable of. The darkest hour may carry within it the dawn of our true direction in life.

C. S. Lewis remarked, "Prostitutes are in no danger of finding their present life so satisfactory that they cannot turn to God: the proud, the avaricious, the self-righteous, are in that danger."[64] Those with chronic or acute pain do not find their present life satisfying, and the resulting sense of dislocation can nudge them into inward change. In removing sufferers from comfortable surroundings, the desert sojourn of the pain experience can enable them to gain a renewed perspective on their lives. Ironically, what seems to have derailed them can point them in new and more meaningful directions. This experience can enlarge their vision, opening them to embrace mystery. As in the desert, with the healing process there is always more than what meets the eye.

ACCEPTING THE MYSTERY OF HEALING

Carl Miller, a patient of mine, formerly was an Olympic weight-lifting coach. Now in his sixties, he lives in Santa Fe, New Mexico. Carl has experienced enormous pain and suffering, and has dealt with it from a spiritual perspective. Carl is on the forefront of the Olympic weight lifting sport. He has earned many U.S. and world records. He is fifty-eight years old. Carl started body-building and weight-training in his early adulthood because he suffered from melancholy. He found that exercise was a powerful way to manage this oppressive condition.

Early in his development of the sport as he lifted progressively increasing weights, Carl sustained several injuries. Eventually, he had to have a spinal fusion; the surgery was performed in Japan and revised in

Chicago. Carl has had thirteen major operations, most of them on his back and musculoskeletal system. He has been able to come back from every operation and reactivate by using small, meaningful goals each day—staying very physically productive and avoiding a limited range of motion.

Facing what Carl did, the average person might have settled for a limited range of motion, dependence on medications, or capitulation to a pain syndrome. Because of his need to treat the melancholy, Carl fought back each time and was able to regain strength and continue to refine his Olympic weightlifting technique. Although he has worked hard physically, Carl feels that the arena of true struggle comprises the psychological and spiritual challenges of overcoming adversity. Exercise has been a gift to him, and he shares it with others in his conditioning-center business. There is something mysterious about what makes a person reach beyond pain to conquer problems, he believes. If we try to hard to analyze it, we can destroy the mystery by dissecting it.

I have found that exclusive reliance on injections, surgery, or medications usually does not produce significant long-term improvement. Nevertheless, if we accept that the healing process is in many respects a mystery and therefore includes spiritual factors along with physical and psychological, we will often witness significant shifts toward wellness. Western healthcare providers are frequently burdened with the thought that the buck stops with them, so if they have neither cured the problem nor relieved the pain, they feel a sense of failure. Native American and Hispanic healers, however, are not as invested in being the most impor-tant part of the healing process. The curandera before Diós and the medicine man before the Great Spirit are human channels of healing, passive vehicles rather than the source itself. Curanderas often pray continuously while attending to their patients. Western physicians might take a cue from them by making the uncomfortable jump of offering prayer for healing their patients. They may find that dethroning themselves as the healer in favor of becoming a helpful vehicle would at times increase their effectiveness.

There are times when healers should leave analysis and procedures on the shelf, at least for a moment, and creatively, lovingly practice prayer for those in pain and suffering. It may be as simple as one phrase: "Help us with the healing." It may be a petitionary prayer such as asking for clear medical judgment or strength to carry on as a healer. It may be the prayer of the forsaken: "Where are you, God, in this struggle to help and to heal?" At times it will simply be the prayer of relinquishment—"Thy will be done"—which leads to the prayer of rest, or a turning over of all fears, worries, and responsibilities to a greater power.

Richard Foster models a wisdom that comes to the healer when he learns to practice prayer that is authentic and unique: "Oh Father, so many hurt today. Help me stand with them in suffering. My temptation is to offer some quick prayer and to send them off rather than to endure with them the desolation and the desert of suffering. Show me the pathway into their pain."[65]

Accepting the mystery of healing involves becoming more receptive to techniques that defy an exact, scientifically verified justification. Studies have shown how critically important touch is to newborn babies. It is not much of a leap to transpose the potential power of touch to adults in pain and fear. In Native American and Hispanic healing cultures, appropriate touch is imperative for treating illness. Certain Christian denominations practice the laying on of hands for healing illness or restoring emotional and spiritual well-being. In alternative healing practices, bodywork treatments such as acupressure and massage have proven remarkably effective in relieving both physical and psychological distress.

Counter-productive to the healing process, we tend to assume we can control pain by increasing our technical sophistication and carefully matching up symptoms to precise diagnoses and corresponding procedures. The sheer anxiety of our rush to eliminate pain by applying the proper technique often makes the pain worse. Fear, anger, loneliness, and helplessness are all pain intensifiers. When a patient arrives in the hospital and the nurses rush in to take blood pressure and the lab technician arrives to draw blood, the patient has no choice but to lie passively in bed being waited upon—often with no clue as to what is being done and why. This scenario breeds the insidious development of helplessness, a pain intensifier. If the patient were instead given tasks or goals as a way of participating in the process of recovery, it could ease the states of mind that are pain intensifiers.

Embracing the mystery of healing can also help us embrace the mystery of illness and suffering. Inevitably we search for cause-and-effect relationships as a way of understanding the painful and bewildering circumstances thrust upon us. Those in severe pain often aggravate their distress with the anxiety of second-guessing: *if only I had changed my diet or exercised more regularly or taken the proper steps right away instead of procrastinating, I might have avoided this.* Religious people especially are prone to becoming tormented by guilt, presuming sin or spiritual failure and feeling condemned by the ultimate authority in the universe: *What did I do wrong? What is God trying to tell me?* This self-flagellation is counter-productive when dealing with pain.

The Bible is sometimes invoked to justify rigid positions on who or what warrants divine favor or disfavor—yet some of its central stories illustrate the profound mystery of illness and suffering. The Old Testament figure Job was subjected to virtually every conceivable form of affliction. His protest to God was met not with explanation but with a thundering reproach of any effort to reduce the ways of the Divine to what could humanly be understood. Those who received the greatest censure in Job's story were the pious religious authorities who presumed to explain God's ways to Job with simplistic cause-and-effect propositions, such as punishment for Job's supposed sins.

In the New Testament, Jesus' disciples questioned him about why a blind man had been afflicted with his illness—whose sin caused it, they asked him, the man's or his parents'? Internalizing the moralistic legalism of the Pharisees, they believed that illness was a sign of God's displeasure. Jesus baffled them by answering that sin had nothing to do with it. It was something God could use to bring good from.

It is very difficult to accept the mystery of pain when it feels like a punishment we don't deserve for a transgression we weren't aware we had committed—or one that was not severe enough to merit such a consequence. Punishment works only when we know the reason behind it and can choose to change our behavior accordingly. Mystery is maddening because there is no way to identify reasons behind events, to make cause-and-effect connections, to understand why. A society that prides itself on analysis and accomplishment is powerless before mystery. That is a huge problem for our collective self-esteem.

In pain treatment, we are frequently humbled by the inadequacy and ineffectiveness of mere technique. Indeed, that is often how our pain centers get referrals from other doctors: conventional treatments have not helped. To make any progress, we are compelled to treat patients in an interdisciplinary way. To identify those who are burdened by the attempt to discover cause-and-effect reasons behind their pain, we listen for the "if only" cue, a phrase which is inevitably a danger sign. "If only I had done this...if only I had not done that...things might be different."

I cannot always determine scientifically what has caused a given disease or a pain situation for my patients. But whenever I can and whenever my patients seem open, I do my best to relieve them of unnecessary guilt. Things happen—some of them good, many of them bad, and most beyond our control. Sometimes we can find a purpose in pain; other times it is not apparent. We may not know the answers in our lifetime. "Life is not always a problem to be solved," Henri Nouwen wisely observed, "but a mystery to be entered into."[66]

Helping patients celebrate the mysteries inherent in pain and suffering seems counter-intuitive. Nevertheless, when these mysteries move them toward healing and wholeness, the celebration no longer seems so paradoxical.

STEPS FOR THE PATH:
CELEBRATE THE PARADOXES

1. *Today, I would rate my general pain level as:*

   0   1   2   3   4   5   6   7   8   9   10
   pain free   excruciating pain

2. *Do you recognize paradox in your pain experience?*

3. *One of the paradoxes of the pain experience is learning to rely on your intuition just when you feel the greatest need to depend on others' advice. Choose an area in which you can affirm your unique identity by greater reliance on your inner knowing. How can you incorporate "listening" in your daily routines?*

4. *The desert experience is a way of discovering simplicity and reordering priorities. Consider how your journey through the desert of pain is an opportunity to take a time-out from "ordinary" life, and write down your thoughts.*

CHAPTER EIGHT

A Life Larger than Pain

This is the great challenge of pain: Will you allow it to debilitate you or will you see it as a catalyst to delve deeper into yourself and your beliefs? Will you allow the emotions to distort your inner sense of the truth, or will you recognize pain as a crucible from which you will emerge stronger than ever?

—MENACHEM MENDEL SCHNEERSON[67]

WHEN I AM DRIVING back and forth between our pain centers in Santa Fe and Albuquerque, forced to keep moving at a rapid pace while maintaining a constant pitch of high intensity, cell phone in hand, call-waiting in effect, fax machines humming at both offices, computer ready for the next session, six different phone numbers where I can be reached, and my schedule crammed beyond available time slots, I am often struck by the ironies embedded in this geographical cluster of different cultures. I think of the Native American sitting on the mesa, watching nature unfold. I see the Tibetan Buddhist sitting in his meditation, allowing life to teach him fundamental lessons. I picture my friend who is a nun at Christ in the Desert Monastery, quiet and reflective in prayer, laboring to help others by taking away their pain and refusing to flee from her own.

For me, the process of being still, of endeavoring to find the rhythm and flow of life, is at loggerheads with the life I must maintain for too many hours of the day. It is very difficult to transition from the zone of high-performance intensity and sophisticated technology to the realm of meditation and prayer. Those who have structured their routines to accommodate the rhythms of the inner life are better prepared for dealing with setbacks and reversals than those who manipulate every last detail of their lives to make sure they waste neither time nor opportunity.

How can we cultivate a sense of wholeness when the demands of life seem to fragment our time and attention? How is it possible for a person to feel whole again when she has irretrievably lost an essential part of herself to injury or illness?

My open-heart surgery in France was a major life event. While my physical heart was undergoing repair, my spirit was undergoing renewal. The wonder of healing is that it has less to do with the mechanics of the body than with the wisdom of the spirit. I now approach my appointments with patients as two-way exchanges, expecting to listen as much as talk. I know that our best work together will be done on a heart-to-heart level.

It is commonly assumed that healing means restoration to the state of health prior to the onset of trauma. Some are fortunate enough to experience a complete recovery from injury or illness. Most are not. I want to affirm, emphatically, that it is possible to live a whole life despite the persistence of physical limitations and frailties. Whatever the body may have lost, the sense of integration acquired through struggle can bind together the ragged and unfinished pieces of our lives in a renewal of meaning and purpose.

The process of quietly finding a way forward through difficult circumstances will often lead to a place in which the heart is at peace. As practical encouragement, I offer the following insights, distilled from years of work my patients and I have done together. These are the lessons of the heart we have learned in the school of pain.

YOUR PAIN IS NOT YOUR DESTINY

When pain strikes, you may feel that if it does not get fixed immediately, it will take over your life. But your pain is not your destiny. It is an affliction that will test you and change you, but it need not dictate your future.

Pain has only as much power over you as you grant it. This lesson has become clear to me especially in the contrast between Anglo and Native American ways of life. I am fortunate to count among my friends a renowned Hopi-Tewa artist named Dan Namingha, who lives near us in Santa Fe.

Dan was raised by his grandfather, a very wise man I was able to meet years ago when Dan was setting the site for his house and studio. I was out on a walk and noticed an elderly man sitting on the hill near our home. As I walked close to him, I could see he was a traditional Hopi Indian. Although he was blind, he sensed my approach. He greeted me and held my hands with his own—old, arthritic, and beautiful—chatting with me in halting English. As I felt enveloped by his deep tender voice and gentle way, our friendship with the Namingha family began.

Dan speaks slowly, with a reflective manner rare in our fast-paced Western culture. He has a patient way of being in the world, a quality of calmness and quietness markedly absent of the ego-driven need to talk loudly enough to ensure that he is heard. I find that hearing what Dan has to say requires careful listening, because he speaks softly with a hypnotic and soothing cadence that lulls me into its rhythms.

Our fear of pain can so preoccupy us that it overwhelms everything else in life and becomes our defining characteristic. Dan explained to me that the Hopi understanding of pain places it on a continuum in the flow of everyday life, an inevitable part of existence. Every day is a healing process. When he arises, he must be joyful and optimistic, always aware of his closeness to the earth and his relationship with all of nature.

Westerners tend to compartmentalize spirituality as one of many dimensions in life, separating it out as a category of life-enhancing potential. We work on our spiritual life to achieve inner well-being in the same way that we go to the health club to achieve physical fitness, or take adult education classes to sharpen mental fitness. This separation is unnatural for the Hopi, according to Dan. Hopis are more likely to say, "I continue to grow and to flow spiritually," in an all-inclusive referral to the totality of their life. Spirituality is integral to the Hopi way of life, from the moment of awakening to every thought and activity throughout the day.

The Hopi practice of dealing with pain involves becoming immersed in herbal medicines and ceremonies. These rituals divert attention from the physical pain and help promote healing by marginalizing the pain and reaffirming the individual's identity in the unified matrix of life—human, natural, and supernatural. This is a powerful ritual involving a communal ceremony of song and dance performed by sacred Hopi societies to clarify one's place in the universe.

WHAT YOU THINK WILL SAVE YOU IS NOT YOUR SAVIOR

When immediate gratification is a core value, interventions such as surgery, narcotics, and nerve blocks take on an inflated importance. In his discussion of whether to treat disc herniation patients with pain pills, surgery, or both, Dr. Frank Vertosick, Jr. describes the I-want-it-now tendency:

> Some people will ask for surgery sooner than others; some people can tolerate pain better than others. I doubt that I would have earned much of a living doing pain surgery in ancient Sparta, but in a community composed largely of type A urban professionals who believe that every shred of their pain should have been gone yesterday, I stay busy.[68]

The very thing you think will save you, however, might possibly be the thing that further entrenches your pain by sending you on an obsessive hunt for an immediate solution. You may find an answer that fulfills its promise temporarily, but you may also be in a circumstance for which no procedure will take the pain away completely. Therefore, the path to a more fulfilling life, away from the limiting constraints of raw pain, leads through many dimensions of the healing process, not just the narrow dimension of pain relief. We tend to be so impatient with anything that derails us from our path toward the good life that we are unwilling or unable to see the opportunities that may be surfacing because of our derailment. Learning to walk the unchosen path requires patience and quiet reflection. It may lead to an opportunity for reclaiming our lost sense of self.

I will never forget a little old man, physically broken, who climbed up onto the operating table with great difficulty. We wheeled him into the operating room, where I was the presiding anesthesiologist. I had just come from a workout at the gym, and my preoccupation with optimal physical health had me mentally reviewing my schedule for the rest of the day to decide how I could fit in a run. This little man looked up at me with twinkling blue eyes, winked and said, "You know, I'm ninety years old, and I'm not much physically, but every day I grow spiritually." His comment pulled me up short—here I was, the all-knowing doctor standing over his patient, compartmentalizing my life to try and add up to a whole person, when the patient had just let slip a little remark more profound than all my planning and scheming. This wizened little man, on his deathbed for all he knew, had discovered what is most important in life—and even more important, how to build his life upon it.

Healing can teach us that our most important growth takes place within. Yes, we need to honor the gift of the body, but as it ages we need to shift our focus in order to continue growing. As physical growth deteriorates, spiritual growth can accelerate. In some cases, the spiritual growth may be what strengthens physical healing because spirit and body are in better balance.

Acute pain, such as what we feel when recovering from surgery, often has a physiological purpose. In these cases I will tell patients that they are going to participate in a miracle: the process of healing. Millions of cells know exactly what to do in a series of processes far more intricate than the most advanced computer functions. The sensations people will feel after surgery are those of healing, and they should try to reframe them as sensations with a positive purpose—not feelings associated with something bad or something they have done wrong.

This kind of thinking is a change from the voices we are used to hearing, which tell us that pain is punishment, illness implies guilt, physical limitations reduce our capacity for a meaningful life, and aging should be feared and resisted. Turn your dread and fear into expectation, looking for teachers where you least expect them. Your own intuition may be one of your greatest sources of wisdom. Learn to respect it, and you will be able to turn a deaf ear to the false voices that speak the loudest. You may well discover the source of your salvation in the wisdom of quiet reflection and spiritual reorientation.

PAIN CAN ENLARGE YOUR LIFE INSTEAD OF SHRINK IT

Chronic pain can invite us to live a larger life than we had planned. More frequently, however, it leads to a constricted life. Some of this is a patient's choice. The challenge of pain can open up new boundaries, but only if we choose to break the cycle by stepping outside it, doing something different to energize ourselves in defiance of the defeat that pain insinuates.

But change is not easy. "Any significant change in one's life is, in its broadest sense, suffering," writes William J. O'Malley. "Growth itself is suffering, since we have to give up a self we were comfortable with in order to evolve into a better self. But we live in an ethos that recoils even from inconvenience—much less the troublesome effort to change one's habits...As Carl Jung insists, 'evading legitimate suffering that comes simply from dealing with the world we were dealt always ends in neurosis—anxiety, obsessions, narcissism, and blaming our faults on our personalities rather than blaming our personalities on our faults.'"[69]

The power to change often begins with the confession of powerlessness. Pain brings us to this threshold with unerring accuracy. It forces us to reckon with our inability to construct our lives according to plan. At first this feels like weakness, which is why so many of us shrink back from crossing this threshold. It is simply too difficult to admit our own power-lessness. Yet there is strength in weakness, because it allows us to exchange the illusion of a powerful self for the truth of an authentic self—a self unfettered by falsehoods and empowered by grace.

In the Christian tradition, power revealed in weakness is a divine paradox. The cross is the ultimate representation of this paradox, but the Bible is replete with stories of how human frailty invokes divine strength. When Jesus was making his way through pressing crowds to visit a dying little girl, a woman who had suffered for years with uncontrollable bleeding approached him from behind—"If I but touch his clothes, I will be made well," she vowed. Aware of this distinct touch amid the jostling and shoving because he felt power flowing out from his body, Jesus immediately turned around to see who it was. When the woman fearfully confessed to him, he responded, "Daughter, your faith has made you well; go in peace, and be healed of your disease."[70]

The divine empowerment is not necessarily physical restoration, however, as the apostle Paul discovered when he begged for deliverance from a tormenting problem, "the thorn in the flesh." Instead of responding as Paul had initially hoped, God gave him a paradoxical gift—the discovery of how grace comes not with the removal of suffering, but in the very experience of suffering itself, "for power is made perfect in weakness."[71]

The "larger life" we can discover through pain is defined not by miraculous restoration of health, but by the marvelous re-envisioning of existence that becomes possible when we face into our struggles instead of turning away from them.

HOPELESSNESS CAN LEAD TO HOPE

Dietrich Bonhoeffer, who died a martyr in the German resistance movement against Hitler, wrote from his prison cell, "it is easier to suffer physical death than the pain of spiritual death."[72] In our fear, suffering looms as the ultimate enemy. But suffering is not fatal, only hopelessness is. Physical pain need not equal hopelessness, but that is the reality for some sufferers.

The good news is that hopelessness can lead to hope. Once all conventional sources of help have been exhausted, the work of the spirit often begins in earnest. This is the path that leads beyond despair to a discovery of something higher and deeper as a source of meaning and purpose. Thus the suffering surrounding an event may be the signal for authentic hope, a harbinger of spiritual awakening and rebirth.

Some people can walk the fragile ground between despair and hope. For others it is too difficult, and they need guidance and support to move beyond hopelessness. One of the missions of the Pain Center is to support those who are struggling for hope by helping them turn their backs on despair.

One of my patients, whom we affectionately dubbed "La Contessa," is from an aristocratic New Mexico family descended from sixteenth-century Conquistadors. When I began treating her several years ago, she was already in her eighties. An elegant and dignified woman, she frequently wore her hair up in a tiara fashion, projecting a sense of social prominence with grace and humility. A deeply spiritual person, she never appeared without her cross and rosary beads. Upon our first meeting, I was stunned to see how contorted her body had become as a result of scoliosis (curvature of the spine) and severe arthritis in her hands and feet. She suffered constant pain, extreme at times, but she seldom manifested that pain through her behavior and rarely complained. In contrast to her deformed limbs, she radiated a joyful spirit through her shining eyes and smiling countenance. There was a power about her that commanded respect—indeed, I knew she was greatly revered by her children, grandchildren, and great-grandchildren.

As so often happens, the patient cares for the caregiver. It was clear from the outset that La Contessa was teaching me a crucial lesson of the heart. What had this lady learned that enabled her to be joyful while enduring virtually continual pain? Now in her nineties, she hardly ever voices discontent even though she is barely able to walk, and she is frequently awake during the night trying to reposition herself to ease the pain. Yet she is always giving to others—to her grandchildren, to her children, to the community, even to her physicians. She will often bring me a plate of *biscochitos*, traditional Spanish cookies.

At long last, I asked La Contessa what enabled her to focus beyond her pain and become such a spirit-filled person.

"For many years now, Dr. Hinds," she replied, "I have realized that my failing body is just a cocoon. It is a chrysalis, which is becoming more rigid and of less value. But the eternal spirit within me is getting ready to become a butterfly, which will emerge and go to eternity."

La Contessa might have spent her time pining wistfully for her youth and outward beauty, which had long since faded. She could easily have yielded to despair over her increasingly crippled and painful body. Instead, she allowed these losses to inspire hope by viewing them as reminders of her coming transformation.

Indeed, La Contessa's transformation has begun already. She has discovered the gift of receiving in the act of giving. She will probably not live much longer, but her joy at the prospect of eternity and the radiance she gives to all those associated with her will linger in our memories when the time arrives for her to take wing.

Those who share La Contessa's belief in heaven—a life after death of blissful union with God in the redemption of earthly life—have a clear goal in which to place their hope. What about those who do not have religious faith? What does hope mean for them? In his description of pain patients who have "successfully coped" with suffering, Philip Yancey offers a very simple definition: "Hope means simply the belief that something good lies ahead. It is not the same as optimism or wishful thinking, for these imply a denial of reality."[73]

Pain patients have already had many hopes ripped out of their grasp. They know all too well what has failed them as a trustworthy source of hope, but they need not live in that failure. They have an opportunity to redefine the "good" in life. I have seen over and over again that those who seek, will find.

EMBRACE MYSTERY WHILE YOU SEEK ANSWERS

Suffering is much easier to philosophize away when it happens to other people. "There's no reason for it; it's just random chance," some will say. "You just don't know where the roulette wheel will stop." The religiously fervent might explain it away as "God's will," implying that God wanted some terrible thing to happen, as if human beings are just pawns on an inscrutable divine chessboard. When suffering hits home, however, the explanations dissolve before the agonizing question, "Why?"

Some pain seems easier to bear if we think we know why it happened, or what purpose it will serve. Even bad answers seem preferable to no answers. The problem is that these "answers" can short-circuit the healing process in a kind of arrested development.

The paradox of pain is likely to take from you the meaning you thought you needed and replace it with a meaning you could not have anticipated. You will never get a satisfactory answer to the plea, "Why is this experience happening to me?" But you may be propelled into a new way of looking at your life with the question, "How is this experience teaching me about what is most important in my life?" If you keep asking the "why" question over and over again, you are likely to become entrenched—because, once again, you have been trapped into focusing on the pain, which will only intensify it. You are faced with a decision: respond to your pain by obsessing over it, or break the cycle by choosing to live with unanswered questions.

Despite my deepest desire for patients to be cured of their illnesses and to recover fully from their injuries, I look beyond the physiological healing for the profound inward healing of the heart. Pain can be the unwanted messenger that nevertheless gets our attention, the harsh teacher who leads us to the most important lessons.

There are times in my work as a healthcare provider when I feel a sense of failure because the pain persists despite all my attempts to alleviate it. Perhaps this is a reminder to be humbled by the knowledge that ultimately I am not in control. It may be an invitation to recognize that alongside my efforts to apply the latest research and the most sophisticated techniques in serving my patients, I must respect the holy ground on which we walk together. My professional drive to diagnose and treat with precision and accuracy must be tempered by the recognition that my patients' healing, and sometimes their injuries as well, involve mysteries beyond the reach of my extensive training and expensive technology.

Native Americans have a wonderful tendency to laugh at Anglo attempts to understand and master everything. Their ready laughter keeps them from taking themselves too seriously—a liability that is perhaps endemic to the medical profession. Native Americans would say that in times of pain there is a lesson to be learned, so look at the lesson the pain is bringing you. If you simply suppress it with medication or a procedure, you run the risk of failing to complete the process of learning whatever it is the pain may be teaching you.

Dan Namingha helped me understand that when you try to dissect the reasons for adversity, you risk destroying the mystery of life and death, and healing and suffering. Embracing the unknown is scary, but there comes a time when that is exactly what you need to do. Turning over your fear and resting in mystery is not a common practice in our society. When my patients go against the grain and accept their difficult circumstances instead of running from them, I see them begin to inhale a deep, refreshing calm. They are letting go of the burden of answers. Some of them shift the burden to God; others let it slide away in meditation as an illusory demand of the ego. Whatever their concept of mystery, embracing it becomes a healing way of responding to pain—a pain modifier.

ACCEPT THE CRUCIBLE OF TRANSFORMATION

Suffering leads to the wisdom of experience. I have found that the wisest spiritual guides tend to be people who have learned to live with pain. They do not spout shallow advice. They speak from the struggle of their own experience, sharing what they have learned firsthand. These individuals model for me a way of walking through darkness, but they cannot learn my lessons for me. The only way I can acquire the wisdom of experience is the hard way.

Suffering exacts a great price, but it can also yield a great return: transformation. "The value of unmerited suffering," observed Martin Luther King, Jr., "[calls us] either to react with bitterness or seek to transform the suffering into a creative force." You may not have the ability to change the circumstances of your suffering, but you do have the ability to choose how you will respond to those circumstances. For some, this choice may be the only path of release. It is not merely a positive-thinking technique, an exercise in the power of the mind. It is, fundamentally, a commitment made on the level of the human spirit—a determination that engages the heart as much as, if not more than, the mind.

Acquiring the wisdom of experience necessitates walking through the crucible of transformation. When you accept instead of resist the lessons waiting there for you, you are doing more than employing a cognitive tool for attitude adjustment. You are ascending on a spiritual level to what may be a powerful transformation within the depths of your being.

All of life is, in a sense, a crucible of inward change if we are willing to harvest our experiences to gain wisdom rather than frittering the experiences away. But suffering can accelerate transformation. People will sometimes comment after a crisis, "I feel as if I have lived several lifetimes through this." That is because they have sustained a crash course in lessons of the heart: what someone else might learn in a four-year program has just been distilled into a month-long summer school intensive.

You would not volunteer for such a course of study. Only the rare few choose to submit themselves to suffering in order to grow from it. The rest of us are dragged into it kicking and screaming. Once you find yourself there, you can either keep kicking and screaming, or you can recognize that pain has placed you in a crucible for transformation. If you allow your suffering to change you instead of harden you, chances are you will not want to go back to being the person you were before the struggle. You will be too grateful for the person it has enabled you to become.

We tend to like surprises, but pain always arrives as an unpleasant and unwelcome surprise. It is an alarm that injury has occurred. After the initial shock, you may find that pain is bringing you a welcome surprise: it is helping your heart find its way back home. You would never have known the injury was there if pain had not revealed it to you. Now you have a chance to do something about it, to choose to move toward healing. Apart from how your body recovers from injury or rallies to fight off illness, the spiritual struggle that pain has pitched you into can open up matters of the heart. You may find that hidden hurts or unacknowledged emotional injuries are now emerging. Pain has revealed what otherwise would have remained dormant, and your heart is beginning to move from aching to healing. That is a transformation we all long for.

WHAT YOU FIND MAY BE WORTH MORE THAN YOU LOST

Most of us think recovery means regaining what was damaged by injury or illness. In living through crisis, you may recover something that had been missing in your life before you sustained injury: perhaps a richer and more satisfying way to live.

"Those who find their life will lose it," Jesus declared, "and those who lose their life for my sake will find it."[74] The search for the good life can lead to an emotional and spiritual dead end if we attach ultimate significance to things that can easily fail us: material possessions, social status, relationships, or a physically comfortable life. Chronic pain or physical disability can make people feel that life as they knew it is over—which, in a sense, it is. They now have to forge a different way of life, and they may find that the new beginning is more significant than what has just ended.

Dr. Frank Vertosick describes this reversal of lost and found in the life of a woman with intractable face pain.

> [She] enjoyed counseling other victims of face pain so much that she began to see her own illness in a different light. Without personally experiencing the disease, she would never have had the opportunity to minister to others. She found meaning in an otherwise meaningless malady and came to see it as a blessing. In a sense, she was cured, not by craniotomy but by a restructuring of her attitude.[75]

The title of Dr. Paul Brand's book, *The Gift of Pain*,[76] captures this paradox. We would not choose to experience physical suffering, but if we have the vision to see them, we may recognize gifts wrapped in the losses. The habit of paying attention to these hidden gifts can help awaken us to the goodness at the heart of life.

Elizabeth O'Connor, author of *Cry Pain, Cry Hope: Thresholds to Purpose*, was a spiritual guide to thousands of people through her writing and in her personal ministry at an inner-city church in Washington, DC. She suffered from severe rheumatoid arthritis, which eventually confined her to a very restricted way of life. She learned to praise God for both her strengths and her weaknesses, to flow with what is inevitable rather than to fight it as a destructive enemy. "Once again the lion and the lamb in me approached each other and they lay down together," she wrote. "I saw how He who had made one had also made the other...As I move closer to the pain inside me, I found myself wanting to be closer to the pain outside of me." O'Connor had decided to be more of a support to a world in pain.

LOOK FOR JOY IN SUFFERING

Whether the crucible of pain leads to a hardening or softening of a person's spirit usually manifests itself in the absence or presence of joy. Certainly there is no joy in the pain itself. But I have observed that those who affirm some kind of spiritual transcendence—a life with meaning beyond earthly pain and suffering, whether now or in the hereafter—discover a joy that has nothing to do with happiness in the conventional sense. Stripped of the comforts that others can afford to take for granted, they are free to discover a life that no longer depends upon their ability to make it happen. It is defined not by what they can acquire, but by what they can receive.

During my thirty-five years in medicine, I felt the most selfless during my tour of duty in Vietnam. One assignment placed me as the commanding officer of a mobile clearing station—like a MASH unit, except not as advanced. At age twenty-six, after just one year of general surgery residency, I was in charge of 160 people: medics, x-ray technicians, and soldiers who protected us. We took in anyone who was injured and did the best we could for them. There were lots of them, every day. We patched up damaged limbs, tried to mend broken bodies, and cursed mortal wounds.

It had been a grim relief for me to go to Vietnam. I had left on bad terms with a woman, and the sense that I had nothing left to lose gave me a devil-may-care attitude. It was frightening nevertheless, and it was constant work. Our remote location removed us from all distractions— no girls, no places to shop, no idle time to kill, and no self-preoccupation. I was able to focus entirely on serving others.

One morning I woke up and realized that I actually felt joyful, because I was able to live each day outside of myself. My mission was simple: take care of as many people as possible, and give everything I could in the effort to do so. I have never captured that sense of selflessness since then, and I have never again tasted quite the same joy.

Feeling good does not necessarily mean feeling joyful. Feeling good will not sustain you in the crises of life. Finding a solution to your pain will not necessarily bring you joy. The surprise in suffering is that it may help you find interludes of joy and peace, which will sustain you when you are not feeling good. My friend Sister Mary Joaquin at Christ in the Desert retreat center, suffering with terrible arthritis, is very clear on the distinction between feeling good and feeling joyful. One is a mental and physical condition; the other is a spiritual reality.

PRACTICE GRATITUDE AMID LOSS

I have a place of retreat in Colorado along the western edge of a mountain pass. The house sits on the bank of the San Juan River in a cleft surrounded by ancient and majestic mountains. I have cultivated the land to help nurture the living things that depend upon it, especially by planting trees. On the north side of the house I am particularly proud of three young ponderosa pines thriving on the rocky slope overlooking the river. They are the surviving remnant of fifty tiny seedlings I planted with great care, investing many hours of time. Visitors inevitably cluck with disappointment over the forty-seven trees that didn't make it, but I feel fortunate to watch these three now becoming a permanent part of the landscape. They remind me to be grateful for the miraculous presence of living things in the vast web of life that connects us all.

One of my patients was a well groomed, middle-aged, matronly woman. Examining her chart, I discovered she was HIV positive. She had a type of neuropathic pain often seen in AIDS patients. She told me that after her first husband died, she remarried. She subsequently found out, while pregnant with her second husband's child, that he was HIV positive. Her daughter is now ten and HIV negative. Her second husband died in 1992 of AIDS. She has now converted from HIV positive to AIDS. She continues to be calm and sweet, with a surprising sense of peace.

While I was performing a risky and painful procedure on her, I felt her peacefulness transmitted to me. When I later told her that it was an honor to help her with her pain, she commented that her situation had become a gift. Through her dark night of the soul, she had grown so much spiritually that she felt she'd been given a glimpse of eternity. This would not have happened, she said, without the devastating diagnosis. Even under such terrible circumstances, she would not choose to go back to where she had been. Although her worry is now for the health of her young daughter, she is grateful for the inward renewal that emerged in her sojourn through deep valleys and her struggle to maintain some degree of health and equanimity.

Loss has a way of forcing us to give up our personal agendas. When we stop making demands for what we want, we will have room to acknowledge what we have.

WHOLENESS COMES THROUGH BROKENNESS

When difficult experiences reveal how incomplete and fragmented our lives are, we confront our vulnerability to confusion and helplessness. We come face to face with our brokenness—not just the broken back, but the broken spirit that cannot deal with the broken back. We mourn the untimely loss of childhood because our intense society does not allow time and freedom to be a child. We live with the bitter failure of an intimate relationship because we have displaced all our energies in striving for the life we thought we needed.

When circumstances force us to examine our incompleteness, it raises the possibility that we can gather these fragments into a whole. The drive toward healing is the recovery from the losses associated with the pain and suffering. As the body strives to overcome injury and recover physical wholeness, spiritually we strive to heal heartache and recover an internal sense of wholeness. When suffering is transformed from meaningless loss to a redefinition of meaning and purpose, wholeness no longer depends on physical health or outward accomplishments. It arises from the recognition that what happens in your heart is more powerful than what happens in your body. It is felt in the inner peace of realizing that external losses can give you a greater awareness of where your life is truly centered. You can meet loss with acceptance, because instead of pulling you apart as you feared, it can help put you back together in a new integration of body, mind, and spirit.

Dr. Rachel Naomi Remen, bestselling author of *Kitchen Table Wisdom*,[78] believes that healing of our fragmented culture will come through the heart. Her focus on giving "blessings" by affirming the goodness and worth of each individual is partly a consequence of her struggle with complications of Crohn's disease, which struck her at age fifteen. This illness, not her medical expertise, has shaped her work of compassion and caring. Her recent book *My Grandfather's Blessing*[79] recounts the spiritual influence of her grandfather, a rabbi, who taught her the importance of connecting with others. "No one has ever said to me 'If I die of this illness, I will miss my Mercedes,'" she observed. "Yet pursuit of the Mercedes has been their whole life." Illness triggers the realization that "what truly matters, at the edge of life, is who we have touched." Dr. Ramen considers her illness a blessing, because it has made her a much wiser person: "I could not do the work I have done had I not had experiences that were terribly painful. If we stand before people with all our strengths, joys, pain, and imperfections, others will not feel alone or ashamed." Her perspective reflects the Jewish tradition that wholeness is achieved through brokenness: "Everything in our lives can be used to serve others. Our strength comes from our wholeness, not from our perfection."[80] A renewed understanding of what it means to be a whole person includes weaknesses as well as strengths, limitations as well as achievements. This understanding can lead to such a strong sense of integration and purpose that many people will declare, quite genuinely, that they would not want to go back to who they were before the onset of illness. There is no turning back; they are too grateful for what they have discovered in the struggle.

If you suffer from chronic pain, you will inevitably confront the pain paradox. The infirmity might not ever go away, or it may take a different physiological form, but the pain may lead you on a journey toward wholeness. May your own lessons of the heart, however costly, become your personal treasure—the pearl of great price you discover while turning over the soil in the field of struggle.

STEPS FOR THE PATH:
PRACTICING RENEWAL

1. *Today, I would rate my general pain level as:*

0   1   2   3   4   5   6   7   8   9   10
pain free   excruciating pain

2a. *To help you assess the progress you have made in breaking the cycle of chronic pain, use the following scale to describe where you are now on the continuum from entrenchment to renewal (a "10" represents the most positive position on the scale).*

0   1   2   3   4   5   6   7   8   9   10
depression   hope for the future

0   1   2   3   4   5   6   7   8   9   10
deactivation   reactivation

0   1   2   3   4   5   6   7   8   9   10
dependency   self-reliance

0   1   2   3   4   5   6   7   8   9   10
doctor-seeking   responsibility for my wellness

0   1   2   3   4   5   6   7   8   9   10
drug-seeking   pursuing alternatives

0   1   2   3   4   5   6   7   8   9   10
deteriorating relationships   renewed relationships

0   1   2   3   4   5   6   7   8   9   10
dormant spirituality   spiritually active

2b. Compare your responses to the chart above with those you indicated on the same chart in chapter two. What has changed, and what has stayed the same?

3. How would you describe your areas of greatest growth?

4. Summarize the new or most helpful insights you have gained for living a life larger than your pain.

ENDNOTES

1. Frank T. Vertosick, Jr., M.D. *Why We Hurt: The Natural History of Pain.* New York: Harcourt, 2000, p. 261.

2. Shannon Brownlee and Joannie M. Schrof. The Quality of Mercy. *US News and World Report,* March 17, 1997, pp. 54-67.

3. A Brief Guide to Pain Medicine. American Academy of Pain Medicine, 4700 W Lake Ave., Glenview, IL 60025.

4. M.H. Becker. A medical sociologist looks at health promotion. *Journal of Health and Social Behavior.* 1993:34 (Mar):1-6.

5. JF Riley et al. Chronic pain and functional impairment: assessing beliefs about their relationship. *Arch Phys Med Rehabil.* 1988 Aug, 69(8):579-582.

6. Terry Teachout. Directly from the Heart. *Time,* November 8, 1999, p. 139.

7. Chippewa song, author unknown.

8. Caroline Myss. *Why People Don't Heal and How They Can.* New York: Harmony/Crown, 1997, p. 12.

9. *Ibid.,* p. 7.

10. *Ibid.,* p. 23.

11. From an interview with Ammachi by Linda Johnson, "Questioning Tradition," *Yoga Journal,* July/August 1997, pp. 23-24.

12. From a personal interview, April 6, 2001. Used by permission.

13. Romans 12:2, New Revised Standard Version.

[14] Robert K. Hudnut. *Meeting God in the Darkness*. Ventura, CA: Regal Books, 1989, p. 229.

[15] RA Sternbach and B Tursky. Ethnic differences among housewives in psychophysic and skin potential responses to electroshock. *Psychophysiology* 1965(1): 241-246.

[16] Pema Chödrön. *When Things Fall Apart: Heart Advice for Difficult Times*. Boston: Shambhala, 1997, p. 12.

[17] Romans 12:2, NRSV.

[18] Tom McNichol. The New Faith in Medicine. *USA Weekend,* April 5-7, 1996, pp. 4-5.

[19] DB Larson et al. Scientific Research on Spirituality and Health: A Consensus Report. Rockville MD: NIHR 1988.

[20] Elizabeth Kübler-Ross. *On Death and Dying*. New York: Scribner, 1969.

[21] Paul Brand, Philip Yancey. *Pain: The Gift Nobody Wants*. Grand Rapids, MI: Zondervan, 1993.

[22] *Ibid.*

[23] *Ibid.*, p. 80.

[24] *Ibid.*, pp. 187-188.

[25] *Ibid.*, pp. 233-234.

[26] Diogenes Allen. *The Traces of God*. np: Cowley, 1981, pp. 48-49.

[27] Chip Brown. *Afterwards, You're a Genius: Faith, Medicine, and the Metaphysics of Healing*. New York: Riverhead/Penguin Putnam, 1998, p. 47.

28 Fordyce, Wilbert. Psychologist at University of Washington Medical School Pain Center, Seattle.

29 Herbert Benson. *Timeless Healing. The Power and Biology of Belief.* Simon and Schuster, 1997.

30 *Ibid.*, p. 20.

31 *Ibid.*, p 34.

32 Viktor E. Frankl. *The Doctor and the Soul,* second ed. New York: Vintage, 1986, pp. xv-xvi.

33 Daniel A. Helminiak. *The Human Core of Spirituality: Mind as Psyche and Spirit.* Albany, NY: State University of New York Press, 1996, see esp. pp. 6, 24-25.

34 Elizabeth Roberts and Elias Amidon. *Prayers for a Thousand Years.* San Francisco: Harper San Francisco, 1999, pp. 50-51.

35 The French Correction. Keynote speech by Dr. Carpentier at American Heart Association convention 1985.

36 Richard Foster. *Celebration of Discipline.* San Francisco: Harper & Row, 1978.

37 John Donne. V. Meditation from *Devotions Upon Emergent Occasions in Seventeenth-Century Prose and Poetry,* 2nd ed. Alexander M. Witherspoon and Frank J. Warnke (eds.), New York: Harcourt Brace Jovanovich, 1963.

38 Andres Dubus. *Broken Vessels.* Boston: David R. Godine, 1992, p. 138.

39 Nancy Mairs. *Ordinary Time: Cycles in Marriage, Faith, and Renewal.* Boston: Beacon Press, 1993, p. 178.

40 Luke 6:21, NRSV.

41 Jeremiah 2:2, NRSV.

42 Gary Zukav. *The Seat of the Soul*. New York: Fireside/Simon & Schuster, 1989, p. 31.

43 Richard Foster. *Prayer: The Heart's True Home*. San Francisco/ Harper, 1964.

44 Zohar, I, 229b.

45 Richard Foster. *Celebration of Discipline*. San Francisco/Harper, 1978.

46 Joseph Sharp. *Living Our Dying*. New York: Hyperion, 1996.

47 Eugene G. d'Aquili and Andrew B. Newberg. *The Mystical Mind: Probing the Biology of Religious Experience*. Minneapolis: Fortress Press, 1999, p. 14.

48 AIDs quilt prayer. Atlanta, GA. www.Aidsquilt.org.

49 Rabbi Harold S. Kushner. American Pain Society Meeting, 1996.

50 A.W. Tozer in *Celebration of Discipline* by Richard Foster. San Francisco/Harper, 1978, pg 54.

51 Allen Diogenes. *The Traces of God*. n.p.:Cowley, 1981, p. 50.

52 Corinthians 12:12, NRSV.

53 Eugene G. d'Aquili and Andrew B. Newberg. *The Mystical Mind: Probing the Biology of Religious Experience*. Minneapolis: Fortress Press, 1999, p. 55.

54 Janet Nyberg, R.N. *Chronic Pain, Finding a Life Worth Living.* New York: Vantage Press, 1994.

55 *Ibid.*, p. 76

56 *Ibid.*, p. 90.

57 *Ibid.*, p. 118.

58 *Ibid.*, p. 126.

59 *Ibid.*

60 John Milton, *Paradise Lost.*

61 Belden C. Lane. *The Solace of Fierce Landscapes.* New York: Oxford University Press, 1998, p. 195.

62 Thomas Merton. *The Wisdom of the Desert.* New York: New Directions Publishing Corp., 1960, p. 3.

63 Pema Chödrön. *Start Where You Are.* Boston: Shambhala, 1994, p. 5.

64 C.S. Lewis. *The Problem of Pain.* New York: Touchstone/Simon & Schuster, 1996, p. 87.

65 Richard Foster. *Prayer: The Heart's True Home.* San Francisco/ Harper, 1964, p. 227

66 Henri Nouwen, JM. *A Cry for Mercy: Prayers from the Genesee.* Orbis Books Reprint Edition, 1994.

67 Menachem Mendel Schneerson. *Toward a Meaningful Life: The Wisdom of the Rebbe,* adap. Simon Jacobson. New York: William Morrow, 1995, p. 128.

68 Frank T. Vertosick, Jr. *Why We Hurt: The Natural History of Pain.* New York: Harcourt, 2000, p. 102.

69 William J. O'Malley. Making Sense of Suffering and Death. *America* 13 April 1996, p. 9.

70 Mark 5:25-34, NRSV.

71 2 Corinthians 12:9, NRSV.

72 Dietrich Bonhoeffer. *Letters and Papers from Prison.* London: SCM Press, 1954.

73 Philip Yancey. *Where is God When It Hurts?* Grand Rapids, MI: Zondervan, 1990, p. 210.

74 Matthew 10:39, NRSV.

75 Frank T. Vertosick, Jr. *Why We Hurt: The Natural History of Pain.* New York: Harcourt, 2000, p. 278.

76 Paul Brand, Philip Yancey. *Pain: The Gift Nobody Wants.* Grand Rapids, MI: Zondervan, 1993, p. 21

77 Elizabeth O'Connor. *Cry Pain, Cry Hope: Thresholds to Purpose.* Waco, TX: Word, 1987, p. 128.

78 Rachel Naomi Remen. *Kitchen Table Wisdom: Stories that Heal.* Riverhead Books, 1977.

79 Rachel Naomi Remen. *My Grandfather's Blessing.* Riverhead Books, 2001.

80 Quoted in "Healing words from a doctor," by Beth Ashley. *Marin Journal*, 5 May 2000.

Recommended Reading

American Academy of Pain Medicine
"A Brief Guide to Pain Medicine"
American Academy of Pain Medicine
4700 W. Lake Avenue, Glenview IL 60025

Anderson, William R. B. and Jesse F. Taylor
Chronic Pain: Taking Command of our Healing
New Energy Press, Minneapolis, 1995

Benson, Herbert , M.D.
Timeless Healing. The Power and Biology of Belief
Simon and Schuster, New York, 1997

Bitman, Barry M.D.
Reprogramming Pain.Transform Pain and Suffering into Health and Success
Ablex Publishing Corporation, Norwood NJ, 1995

Bonhoeffer, Dietrich
Letters and Papers from Prison
SCM Press, London, 1954

Bonica, John J.
The Management of Pain
Lea and Febiger, Philadelphia, 1990

Brand, Dr. Paul with Philip Yancey
Pain: The Gift Nobody Wants
Zondervan, Grand Rapids MI, 1993

Brand, Dr. Paul with Philip Yancey
The Gift of Pain
Zondervan, Grand Rapids MI, 1997

Brena, Steven
Pain and Religion: a Physiological Study
Charles C. Thomas, Springfield IL, 1972

Bresler, Dr. David E. with Richard Trubo
Free Yourself from Pain
Simon and Schuster, New York, 1979

Chaitow, Leon
The Book of Natural Pain Relief
Harper Paperbacks, New York, 1995

Chödrön, Pema
When Things Fall Apart. Heart Advice for Difficult Times
Shambhala Publications, Inc., Boston, 1997

Cycles of Life (from the American Indians)
Editors of Time-Life Books, Alexandria VA, 1994

Dossey, Larry, M.D.
Healing Words. The Power of Prayer and the Practice of Medicine
Harper San Francisco, 1993

Dossey, Larry, M.D.
Prayer is Good Medicine
Harper San Francisco, 1996

Dossey, Larry, M.D.
"In Praise of Unhappiness"
Alternative Therapies, vol 2, no 1; Jan. 1996

Doyle, Derek, Geoffrey W.C. Hanks, and Neil MacDonald
Oxford Testbook of Palliative Medicine
Oxford University Press, Inc., New York, 1993

Feinberg, Steven D., M.D.
"The Pain Medicine Specialist as a Physician-Healer"
The Clinical Journal of Pain, 12:5; 1996

Foster, Richard J.
Prayer. Finding the Heart's True Home
Harper San Francisco, 1964

Friedman, Aleen M.
Treating Chronic Pain. The Healing Partnership
Plenum Press, New York and London, 1992

Hendler, Nelson H., Donlin M. Long, and Thomas N. Wise
Diagnosis and Treatment of Chronic Pain
John Wright, Littleton MA, 1982

Wolff, Helen and Kurt Wolff
Hour of Gold, Hour of Lead
Harcourt Bruce Jovanovich, New York, 1973

Johnsen, Linda
"Questioning Tradition. An Interview with Ammachi"
Yoga Journal; July/August 1997

Kaplan, Marty
"Ambushed by Spirituality"
Time; June 24, 1996

Levin, Carol Lynne
"Tribal Values and Western Medicine"
Native Peoples, vol 10, no 4; Summer 1997

Liptak, Karen
North American Indian Medicine People
Franklin Watts, New York, 1990

Meinhart, Noreen T.
Pain—A Nursing Approach to Assessment and Analysis
Appleton-Century-Crofts, Norwalk CT, 1983

Moyers, Bill
Healing and The Mind
Doubleday, New York, 1993

Myss, Caroline, Ph.D.
Why People Don't Heal and How They Can
Harmony Books, a division of Crown Publishers, Inc., New York, 1997

Nyberg, Janet
Chronic Pain. Finding a Life Worth Living
Vantage Press, New York, 1994

O'Connor, Elizabeth
Cry Pain, Cry Hope. Thresholds to Purpose
World Books, Waco TX, 1987

O'Malley, William J.
"Making sense of suffering and death"
America; 13 April 1996

Perrone, Bobette, H. Henrietta Stockel, and Victoria Krueger
Medicine Women, Curanderas, and Women Doctors
University of Oklahoma Press, Norman OK, 1989

Ross, Dr. A.C.
Mitakuye Oyasin: "We are all Related"
BEAR, Kyle SD, 1989

Schiedermayer, David, M.D.
Putting the Soul Back in Medicine
Baker Books, Grand Rapids MI, 1994

Schlink, Basilea
The Blessings of Illness
Creation House, Carol Steam IL, 1973

Sharp, Joseph
Living our Dying
Hyperion, New York, 1996

Tan, Siang-Yang, PhD
Managing Chronic Pain
InterVarsity Press, Downers Grove IL, 1996

Trotter, Robert T. II and Juan Antonio Chavira
Curanderismo. Mexican American Folk Healing
University of Georgia Press, Athens GA, 1981

Wall, Dr. Patrick D. and Mervyn Jones
Defeating Pain. The War Against a Silent Epidemic
Plenum Press, New York and London, 1991

Yancey, Philip
Where is God When It Hurts?
Zondervan, Grand Rapids MI, 1977

Yancey, Philip
The Jesus I Never Knew
Zondervan, Grand Rapids MI, 1995